Childness and the Myth of the Unfinished Human

Richard Hain

Childness and the Myth of the Unfinished Human

End of Life Medical Ethics in Children

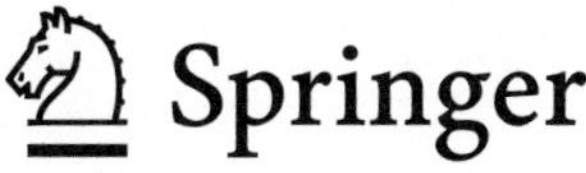 Springer

Richard Hain
All-Wales Paediatric Palliative Care Network
Noah's Ark Children's Hospital
Cardiff, UK

ISBN 978-3-032-12110-3   ISBN 978-3-032-12111-0   (eBook)
https://doi.org/10.1007/978-3-032-12111-0

This Springer imprint is published by the registered company Springer Nature Switzerland AG
The registered company address is: Gewerbestrasse 11, 6330 Cham, Switzerland

If disposing of this product, please recycle the paper.

Dedicated to my ceaselessly loving, kind and funny brother-in-law, David 'Jolyon' Weare (1960–2024), who enjoyed being alive more than anyone else I know despite his profound cognitive impairment, and who taught me a great deal.

Acknowledgements

To all those with whom I have crossed verbal swords in issues concerning ethics in children. You have forced me to reason more carefully than a busy clinician usually has time to do.

To Professor Bob Macauley, who read an earlier manuscript and whose wise and experienced advice has improved the final product out of all recognition.

To my grown-up children, Rebecca, Katherine and Mike, who have teased me about disappearing into my office to write, but have always done it kindly.

Most of all, to my wife Leonie, whose never-failing love, affirmation, support and capacity for celebration have made our lives together a joy. 'He who finds a wife finds what is good' (Prov 18:22a, New International Version).

About the Book

This book begins with the claim that contemporary bioethics is built upon a pervasive and unacknowledged prejudice: that to be fully human is to experience the world as adults do. Philosophers have constructed moral theories that take the cognitive and emotional capacities of adults as the standard for personhood, and used those same theories to evaluate who fall outside that standard. Like a poorly trained algorithm, such an ethic recognises some forms of humanity but fails to notice others. Infants and children—whose ways of perceiving and enjoying existence differ from, rather than falling short of, those of adults—are at risk of being undervalued in moral reasoning and clinical decision-making.

The book traces how adult-normativity has become woven into consequentialist and principlist bioethics, and how that has shaped medicine's language of value. Drawing on philosophy and empirical evidence from developmental psychology and neuroscience, the book argues that childness—the distinctive manner in which infants and children experience their existence—is as authentically human as adultness. An age-neutral bioethic, it proposes, would begin, not with the assumption that being adult is the moral norm, but with the recognition that all distinctively human ways of living and meaning-making are inherently valuable.

Contents

Chapter 1
Introduction

In 2019, researchers made the surprising observation that some autonomous cars are racist. The algorithms on which autonomous vehicles' decision-making is based mean that the cars are less likely to recognise (and so less likely to avoid hitting) a pedestrian whose skin is dark than one whose skin is light.[1]

At first, people wondered if the reason was a technical one: that the car's visual systems made it more difficult for it to register darker skin tones when the light was low. But no—irrespective of the prevailing lighting conditions, it turns out that the car is simply less likely to recognise an obstacle in its path as a pedestrian if the face is dark, so that if forced to choose it is more likely to kill a non-white than a white person. The reason, it appears, is that in teaching the car what a pedestrian looks like, its human developers have chosen to use characteristics that are more common in white than in non-white people. Presumably, although the research does not say so, the developers were working in a culture in which white people are the majority, so that on some probably subconscious level they thought of the characteristics of white people as normal or usual for all people. Perhaps, too, it was partly because they themselves were white.

Of course, this is not, as it were, *real* racism, in the sense that it is not the result of malice on the part of the artificial intelligence that guides the vehicle, or even on the part of its developers. A car's willingness to value the life and health of a white person over that of a black person does, however, represent a form of built-in bias— a prejudice whose origin is ultimately to be found in certain unnoticed prior assumptions. Its developers teach artificial intelligence to avoid killing pedestrians, and on the basis of what it has been taught the car emerges with a clear idea of what it thinks a pedestrian looks like. The more someone diverges from that 'norm', the greater the risk that artificial intelligence will fail to accord that individual his or her proper status as a pedestrian whom the car should avoid hitting.

---

[1] Benjamin Wilson, Judy Hoffman, and Jamie Morgenstern, 'Predictive Inequity in Object Detection', (2019).

Skin colour is not the only arbitrary prejudice to which artificial intelligence is heir. Facial recognition systems are less reliable, for example, when it comes to identifying female faces rather than male faces. It appears that the way developers believe that the normal human is not only white, but also male.[2] But the way in which artificial intelligence undervalues people who are non-white or female pales by comparison with the extent to which it undervalues children. An autonomous vehicle is much more likely to prefer to hit a child than an adult. Again, that is because it is more likely to fail to recognise a child as a pedestrian. The shape of a child is different from what the vehicle has been taught is usual for human beings. She is too small, and the proportions are all wrong. Of course, in reality, those characteristics have no plausible relevance to whether or not the car should choose to hit the child rather than an adjacent adult. But the car's artificial intelligence has been schooled to believe that there is a normal way for pedestrians to be, and it is aware that a child is emphatically not it. The result of that built-in prejudice is that, when it comes to sharing the streets with autonomous cars, the lives of children are given less value than the lives of adults for reasons which reflect prior assumptions that are ultimately arbitrary and have no basis in objective truth.

The 'big idea' in this book is that philosophers have codified a bias against children in moral theories for doctors in much the same way that software developers have codified it in artificial intelligence algorithms for cars. That is, philosophers have developed moral theories that start with certain assumptions about what a normal human person is like. On the basis of those theories, they have gone on to draw conclusions about the value of humans who diverge from those assumed norms, including and perhaps especially children. Those first assumptions are influenced by the culture in which the philosophers have lived, and by the nature of the philosophers themselves.

A philosophical parallel to the idea that children are not pedestrians because of their shape is the idea that they are not persons because of the way they experience and perceive their own existence. Just as developers can introduce systematic bias into an artificial intelligence algorithm by arbitrarily restricting the criteria for 'pedestrianhood', so moral philosophers can introduce it into an ethical theory by arbitrarily restricting the criteria for personhood. Such a restriction is the inevitable result of assuming that the way in which children (particularly infants, for reasons that will become clear later) experience and appreciate their existence is in some way inherently less valuable, or less important, or less *human*, than the way in which adults experience and enjoy *their* living. If you personally are drawn to ratiocination and abstract moral analysis and are living in a culture that takes for granted that the main point of children is to become adults, then it would be natural for you to assume that the characteristics of rational adults are the standard by which the value of all humans should be measured. But unless that can be shown to be objectively true, it is arbitrary and prejudicial and poses a serious risk that the existence

---

[2] Joy Buolamwini and Timnit Gebru, 'Gender Shades: Intersectional Accuracy Disparities in Commercial Gender Classification', *Proceedings of Machine Learning Research,* 81 (2018), 1–15.

of some human beings will be undervalued through systematic bias. An anthropology that considers moral status to rely on a capacity for analytical reason already represents a judgement that the state of being an adult is in some way inherently more valuable than the state of being an infant. Unless we can show that infants and children do not experience or enjoy existence at all—and (spoiler alert) they certainly do—then it is not obvious on the face of it that there is anything especially valuable about experiencing the world as an adult rather than as a child.

I am not, of course, the first person to want to call into question the basic assumption that experiencing existence as a child is less valuable than experiencing it as an adult. It is 2000 years since Jesus suggested that there are ways in which adults should aspire to a child's way of seeing things, rather than simply leaving it behind as they get older.[3] William Blake considered the way adults see things to be frankly inimical to the task of constructing a narrative of the universe, fettering imagination with 'mind-forg'd manacles'—responses catechistically learnt that prevent most adults from observing truths that children can still see.[4] Hans Christian Andersen's story of the emperor's new clothes draws attention to the danger of restricting the way we see and interpret the world to the way in which adults do it, and Pablo Picasso is said to have remarked: 'Every child is an artist. The problem is how to remain an artist once we grow up.'[5] Some philosophers, too, have objected. Ethicist John Wall protests that:

> Children are a third of all humanity. Yet all too often children are considered merely undeveloped adults, passive recipients of care, occupying a separate innocence, or, perhaps, in need of being civilized. Across diverse societies and cultures, and throughout history and today, serious questions of human being, purposes, and responsibilities have usually been considered chiefly from the point of view of adulthood. Childhood has had to borrow its senses of meaning and humanity from those thought to embody them in some fuller, more advanced, or more important way.[6]

---

[3] "At that time the disciples came to Jesus and asked, "Who, then, is the greatest in the kingdom of heaven?" He called a little child to him, and placed the child among them. And he said: "Truly I tell you, unless you change and become like little children, you will never enter the kingdom of heaven. Therefore, whoever takes the lowly position of this child is the greatest in the kingdom of heaven. And whoever welcomes one such child in my name welcomes me. "If anyone causes one of these little ones—those who believe in me—to stumble, it would be better for them to have a large millstone hung around their neck and to be drowned in the depths of the sea." Matt 18:1–6 (New International Version).

[4] "Blake … [has] the child articulate a counterstatement that directly addresses the "one-sided and gloomy official seriousness" of the adult world. His answer to his own question is subversive rather than doctrinal, implicitly confronting the authority claimed by his pastors, masters and parents with an image of the creator not as the Almighty Father but as himself childlike: "He is called by thy name/For he calls himself a Lamb/He is meek & he is mild/He became a little child:/I a child & thou a lamb,/We are called by his name." A. Richardson, 'The Politics of Childhood: Wordsworth, Blake, and Catechistic Method', *ELH-Engl. Lit. Hist.,* 56/4 (1989), 853–68 p. 863.

[5] Quoted in Laurence J. Peter, *Quotations for our time* (London: Souvenir, 1996).

[6] John Wall, *Ethics in light of childhood* (Washington, D.C.: Georgetown University Press, 2010), p. 1.

Wall uses the same term 'humanity' here in two rather different senses. In the first, it denotes all humankind; everyone who belongs to the species *Homo sapiens*. That seems uncontentious; no one seriously doubts that children are human. In the second, however, humanity represents something more numinous: the way of appreciating and experiencing one's existence that is associated with being human. Wall's point is that humanity in that sense has become restricted. It has come to mean only a subset of those ways, namely, the ways in which adults experience their existence. Instead of being recognised as an alternative way of being human, the way in which children appreciate and experience their existence has to derive its value by reference to that adult subset.

Exploring an anthropology of children is complicated by vocabulary (we shall see later, for example, how possessive pronouns can introduce important ambiguities into moral relationships). Contemporary moral philosopher David Archard argues that a clear distinction needs to be made between the state of existing that the word 'childhood' denotes—what it is to exist as a normal human who is not an adult—and the stage of childhood—that is, the period during which a human has not been alive for very long. The stage of being an adult follows that of being a child, but there seems to be no obvious reason why that fact should be relevant to how the two states are valued. Yet, for most of history, philosophy has assumed that the difference is a sound reason for evaluating the state of being a child by reference to the state of being an adult.[7]

As a result, moral theorists have often found themselves having to concede that their theory cannot easily explain inherent value in existing as a child. They have had to conclude either that the child has no value of her own (her value is simply the value that adults ascribe to her) or that the value of being a child needs to be explained by some kind of codicil or exception to the theory. There are perhaps three broad ways in which an adult might be willing to ascribe that kind of value to a child. One is the kind of value she might give to a possession. The second is the kind of value she might accord to an individual who is, as it were, training to become an adult. That merely states the obvious; it is self-evident that if we value individuals because they possess certain qualities, such as reason, then logically we must value any being who demonstrates those qualities, whether a child or not. That succeeds in explaining inherent value in children to the extent that children resemble adults, but it does not challenge the fundamental premise that it is better to exist as an adult than as a child.

---

[7]"How exactly might conceptions of childhood differ? One fundamental line of division lies between thinking of childhood as a *state* and thinking of it as a *stage*. This is the distinction between viewing children as 'being' and as 'becoming'. On the former conception, childhood is a free-standing, independently defined condition; it is not adulthood but its character is not exhausted by this privative fact. On the latter conception childhood occupies a place, or level, within a broader narrative and derives its significance from that narrative—more especially from what succeeds or supplants childhood in the longer story; childhood is not *yet* adulthood and derives much, if not all, of its character from this fact." David Archard, 'The Oxford Handbook of Practical Ethics', in Hugh LaFollette (ed.), (Oxford: Oxford University Press, 2005), p. 92.

The third idea is that we should value a child because he or she will (probably) one day become an adult. That accords some inherent value to existing as a child, because the capacity to become an adult in the fullness of time is part of the nature of being a child now. But it does not succeed in explaining why the value of the infant or child in the present moment should be *the same* as that of the adult he or she might hypothetically become in the future. Nor does it challenge the fundamental idea that ultimately the way in which the normal adult appreciates and engages with her existence in the world is somehow inherently to be preferred over the way in which an infant does so. This 'promissory note' account of a child's value, too, expresses the value of existing as a child largely in terms of the value of being an adult.

Even where they wish to assert that a child has value, many moral theories find themselves endorsing the same problematic idea that the inherent value of existing as an adult is greater than that of existing as a child. That matters in medical ethics, because unless it can be justified on the basis of observable evidence it represents the same sort of arbitrary systematic bias that leads an autonomous car to prefer to kill a child, or a woman, or someone whose skin is dark. A theory that assumes that the most valuable way for humans to experience living is the way that an adult does it has already relegated any other way of doing so to something less valuable. Any moral theory that privileges being an adult over being a child has already made assumptions that we should be able to rely on philosophy to test and to interrogate.

The risk of basing moral reasoning on an unsound first premise is particularly great for consequentialist moral theories. Consequentialism, and particularly utilitarian consequentialism, has historically provided a valuable 'lens' through which to examine medical ethics. There are ways in which it has broadened medicine's understanding of value, making clear that there is a difference between optimising the enjoyment an individual might have in his or her existence in the present moment on the one hand and on the other preserving life at all costs, almost as though life were an abstraction whose value were separable from the value of the person who holds it. That allows a nuanced distinction that was impossible in the past between valuing a living individual and merely valuing the life that that individual holds. But at the same time, a consequentialist approach to bioethics relies heavily on accurately assessing, and correctly evaluating, the characteristics of the individual to whom moral action is being done. While consequentialist theories are able to distinguish between the value of a living individual and the value of that individual's life, they can also easily obscure that difference if they define too narrowly the range of ways in which a being can enjoy his or her existence. If, for example, a particular consequentialist theory starts by asserting that an individual's capacity to enjoy existence primarily expresses their hope that they will continue to live tomorrow, then it has already excluded infants from the community of 'beings who matter' without any reference to whether there might be other equally valid ways in which humans can enjoy existence, some of which the infant might be able to do. There is, in other words, a risk of wrongly ascribing greater consequentialist value to some ways of existing than to others, and the infant and child are particularly vulnerable because they diverge so markedly from the more usual way in which humans enjoy their existence. Furthermore, after that first false step, consequentialist theories can be difficult to critique because they are 'pulling themselves up by their own logical bootstraps'. In order to remain internally consistent, they must systematically disregard values that are not explained on the terms the theorists themselves have set out. But once the assumption has been made that a certain way of experiencing existence is better than any other way of doing it, the theory easily becomes self-fulfilling.

The risks are somewhat less in theories that vest moral value in something other than outcome alone. Principlism, or the 'four principles approach', has dominated the landscape of medical ethics ever since it was first formulated in the late 1970s. It is a practical guide to medical ethics, designed to help clinicians faced with ethical quandaries in practice to consider those quandaries in the light of many different moral theories. Because it draws on deontological and virtue ethics theories (among others) as well as utilitarian consequentialism, the risk of undervaluing children is somewhat mitigated. For those who take the deontological view that there is an obligation on the moral agent to accord equal value to all humans, irrespective of age, the need to explain the inherent value of an individual infant or child does not arise. A doctor will treat a baby as though the baby had the same value as an adult *because it is her obligation to do so*; it does not depend on anything objective about the baby himself. Similarly, those who take a virtue ethics view that what matters morally is being a good person might conclude that they should treat babies and adults with equal respect without needing to know anything about the ways in which either experiences existence.

Because it draws on non-consequentialist as well as consequentialist theories, Principlism is able to conclude with some confidence that doctors and nurses should treat their patients with equal respect, regardless of their age. The grounds for that confidence, however, are not always clear or persuasive because, on the whole, Principlism does not question the fundamental assumption that existing as a child is less valuable than existing as an adult. It asserts that a moral agent should concern herself with an infant's interests, but the basis of that obligation is relationships that are difficult to define except in terms of each other. Principlism asserts that an obligation to respect autonomy should not lead the doctor to ascribe less value to those who lack autonomy, but the basis for that prohibition is essentially that most people today would find such a move repugnant; it is not clear why Principlism's authors feel people would be correct to feel such repugnance. Principlism asserts in the name of justice that children should be considered part of the community of moral actors, but the basis of that participation is largely the capacities they share with adults. The protection that Principlism offers to infants and children, in other words, is through assertions about the way adults are and the way adults should behave; it is not a response to anything inherently valuable about the nature of the child herself. Even in Principlism, there is little attempt to challenge the assumptions that underlie a traditional moral anthropology of children and childhood.

The first step to avoid inadvertently programming bias into autonomous cars would be to ensure that the car is aware of everything it should be looking for. That is, ensuring the car knows every way in which something can be a pedestrian; the sort of object that it should avoid hitting. If it recognises only a subset of those ways, there will inevitably be blind spots and the car will conclude wrongly that there are some people it need not avoid. In order to avoid programming bias against children into a system of bioethics, any theory that is concerned with improving the existence of humans must acknowledge all the ways in which a human can enjoy her existence. If it acknowledges only a subset of those ways, there will inevitably be blind spots and the theory will conclude wrongly that there are some people with whose interests the moral agent need not concern herself.

There are innumerable ways in which humans' lives can be enriched and therefore innumerable ways in which the moral agent can act correctly in order to facilitate another's flourishing. It would be impossible to set out exhaustively what they all are. The idea of 'biographical narrative', however, offers a reasonable and practical approximation. The term describes a distinctively human way in which individuals appreciate and engage with the universe around them. It is a process of constructive meaning-making that ceaselessly solicits new information and builds it into hypotheses that account for what is perceived. We know from empirical research in neurodevelopment psychology that even newborn infants are capable of such constructive narrative, and we are as sure as we can be within the limitations of modern technology that they are actively engaged in doing so. Infants and young children enjoy their existence, albeit in ways that are quite different from the ways in which adults do. It would be a false first step to assume that the only way humans' existence can be improved is by making it more like the way in which an adult enjoys her existence, or by ascribing greater moral value to characteristics such as rationality, independence or futurity that do not characterise the nature of the child.

Even if it were armed with an encyclopaedic knowledge of all the ways in which an object might be a pedestrian, a car might still wrongly evaluate something as a non-pedestrian if it is wrong about what it 'believes' are facts. Pedestrians do not have blue faces, and on those grounds it would be reasonable to tell the car that, if necessary, it should choose to hit the object with the blue face. But that will only work if the car's cameras are switched on and it has been taught correctly that a certain colour is what the developers mean by 'blue'. If the car is to avoid misclassifying children as non-pedestrians, it is important that what it thinks is true is congruent with what is actually true. A bioethicist armed with an encyclopaedic knowledge of all the ways in which a human might be a person might still wrongly evaluate someone as a non-person if the bioethicist is misinformed. Much of what has been published about ethics in infants and children, especially around infanticide, suggests that at the time of writing its authors had little access to empirical evidence about the way in which infants and children actually experience their existence. For most of history, that was because the knowledge simply didn't exist; research had yet to uncover it. That is no longer true and, while many mysteries remain, we are in a much better position than previous generations to establish as a matter of observed fact the ways in which even very young children appreciate and enjoy the business of existing. On the basis of the evidence, my argument will be that a bioethical theory is wrong in the value it ascribes to children is based on a belief that children are incapable of meaningfully enjoying their existence, or if it suggests that the way in which they do so is in some way inherently lacking in value relative to the way in which adults enjoy their existence.

The next task is to consider what medical ethics would look like if we take an approach that considers child and adult to be of equal value, so that we need not evaluate the characteristics of being a child by reference to the way an adult experiences existence. Principlism's four themes can be relatively easily specified to the special case of a human with the cognitive characteristics of a child. The implications of such age-neutral ethical reasoning on exclusively consequentialist bioethical theories, however, are more radical. Some contemporary utilitarian theorists are deeply committed to the idea that the cognitive characteristics of the infant are of such little moral relevance that the moral agent need not concern herself even with whether or not the infant continues to exist. Looking through an age-neutral lens reveals that to be a statement of systematic bias that reflects the theorist's personal (though perhaps unconscious) preference for experiencing existence as an adult, rather than anything rooted in objective truth.

The moral reasoning that leads to age neutrality can usefully be applied to the case of children whose brains have been damaged. Without assuming too narrow a range of ways in which persons can appreciate and enjoy their existence, there is no reason to assume that the way most individual children with cognitive impairment enjoy it is any less inherently valuable than the way in which an ideal adult would do so. On that basis, it is clear that medical decisions over children whose cognition is impaired cannot be made simply on the basis that they belong to a category of patients from whom certain interventions can or should be withheld or withdrawn. That does not commit paediatricians to the position that cognitive impairment is irrelevant to decision-making, or that any child's life should be prolonged for as long as possible. The net balance of an intervention's harm and benefit to the individual child, considered as broadly as possible to include existential as well as biological interests, should guide decision-making, just as it would in a child whose cognition is unimpaired.

Since the way we explain personal value in children will be the central theme of this book, it is important to be clear what we mean by the term 'value'. It is often used to refer to some numinous idea of what a person is worth. That seems to me correct as far as it goes, but is perhaps too vague to be of help in attempting a rational account of personal value. We might consider personal value to be connected to ideas of duty. Humans should perhaps value other humans simply because they are human, and we have certain obligations to others of the same species. Parents should perhaps value children because that kind of obligation represents what it means to be a parent. But the logical relationship between an individual's value, and an agent's duty to care, is ambiguous. Does a moral agent have a duty to care for someone because that is the correct response to that person's inherent value? If so, then an account of her inherent value is in some way logically prior to one of duty, and we are still left needing to explain where it came from. Or does she have value because moral agents have a duty to care for her, a duty that flows from some other source, so that personal value is a logical *consequence* of the moral agent's duty, rather than its source? If so, then the concept of a duty to care is prior to a concept of value, and we are left needing to show what the source of that duty is. Either way—whether we see duty as an expression of value or value as an expression of duty—we find ourselves needing to identify some source of value that is more fundamental than either.

Modern utilitarian consequentialist philosophers, in an effort to pin personal value down to something specific and commensurable, might express personal value, insofar as it relates to bioethics, solely in terms of an individual's capacity to benefit from a certain moral action.[8] It is meaningless, they might argue, for a moral agent to concern herself with consequences to an individual that do not in fact cause that individual benefit or harm. But, while the impact of moral action on others is clearly important, considered as the only contributor to personal value it seems implausibly restrictive. The capacity of a dead person to be harmed by being kicked, for example, is precisely the same as that of a football; but surely it does not follow that in reasoning morally the agent is entitled to ascribe the same value to them both. The consequences of moral action must surely matter, but it does not follow that they are the only thing that matters.

In this book, I will consider an individual's value to mean *the extent to which a moral agent should concern herself with that individual's interests*.[9] The definition is, I hope, sufficiently informative to avoid being vacuous, but it avoids sacrificing breadth on the altar of precision. Expressing value in terms of the obligation it places on the agent does not commit itself to any one particular explanation for the *source* for value, and so avoids an overly meagre or restricted conception of what an individual might consider to be important or what might enable her to flourish. Concern for the interests of a patient with a curable condition should usually manifest itself in vigorous efforts to identify and treat the cause. But the same degree of concern for the interests of a patient whose death is inevitable might easily manifest in rescuing him from fruitless interventions so that he is as comfortable as possible while he dies. Death militates wholly against the interests of the first patient. But it is rather less against the interests of the second, so that there is a real sense in which the moral agent has valued the deaths (and therefore the biological lives) of the two patients differently. According to the definition I have given, however, the two patients themselves have been valued equally highly because the agent's obligations are to concern herself equally with the interests of both.

---

[8] For the purposes of this book, I will consider bioethics to concern how humans should behave towards all living organisms (including themselves), while medical ethics relates specifically to how doctors and other healthcare professionals should behave towards patients.

[9] Some would describe the moral agent's concern for the interests of others as 'compassion'. I have largely avoided using the term in this book. That is not because it is unimportant. Rather the reverse; since it underpins a concern for the interest of others, compassion should, it seems to me, be the basis for any credible system of ethics. But use of the term is inconsistent and it is easily confused with closely related ideas, such as altruism or empathy. For a detailed exploration of the nature and practice of compassion in healthcare, see Joshua Hordern, *Compassion in Healthcare* (Oxford: Oxford University Press, 2020). and Rodger Charlton (ed.), *Compassion* (London: Royal College of General Practitioners, 2015).

To sum up, my argument in this book will be that, just as the value of a human adult's cognition relates to the extent to which it enables her to flourish as an adult, so the value of a human infant's cognition relates to the extent to which he can flourish as a human infant. Such value does not need to rely on how well her cognition equips her to function as an adult, or as a possession of adults, or as some kind of apprentice or incomplete adult. Along the way, I will consider how principlism and various consequentialist approaches to bioethics might look in the light of a moral anthropology that accords equal value to existing as an adult and existing as an infant or child.

Bibliography

Archard D. In: LaFollette H, editor. The Oxford handbook of practical ethics. Oxford: Oxford University Press; 2005.

Buolamwini J, Gebru T. Gender shades: intersectional accuracy disparities in commercial gender classification. Proc Mach Learn Res. 2018;81:1–15.

Charlton R, editor. Compassion. London: Royal College of General Practitioners; 2015.

Hordern J. Compassion in healthcare. Oxford: Oxford University Press; 2020.

Peter LJ. Quotations for our time. London: Souvenir; 1996.

Richardson A. The politics of childhood: wordsworth, blake, and catechistic method. ELH-Engl Lit Hist. 1989;56(4):853–68.

Wall J. Ethics in light of childhood. Washington: Georgetown University Press; 2010.

Wilson B, Hoffman J, Morgenstern J. Predictive inequity in object detection; 2019. https://doi.org/10.48550/arXiv.1902.11097.

Chapter 2
Valuing Children: The Ambivalence of Adults

A visitor to Earth from another planet might find herself perplexed by the personal value that human society ascribes to children. She would soon discover, of course, that individual adults usually care deeply for their own children. She would find a whole mythology of parenthood consisting in accounts of how parents, and particularly mothers, have sacrificed everything for their child. And it would not take much observation for her to realise that those myths are rooted in something about human communities that is real and the everyday experience of many. She would encounter countless parents today who have given up a career in order to care for their child, or who took up a job they disliked in order to give their child the chance of a better life, or even who were willing to risk their own life in order to save that of their child. Such a visitor might also note with interest that the concern adults have for children is not limited to their own offspring. For many adults, the sight of any newborn baby or young child elicits an instinctive, almost visceral, response to cherish and protect.

But there are other observations which, in the interests of unbiased reporting, such a visitor might need to make in her report to Galactic Central Office. The human world, she would have to concede, is run by adults, largely *for* adults. The place of children in it is essentially conditional on how individual adults choose to value them. A liberal society finds it intolerable that we should accord certain groups of adults less value than others more or less on a whim, but its indignation does not extend to rejecting the idea that children's value might be subjective in the same way. We adults cherish our own children, and even coo over other people's, but as a society we seem to be generally comfortable with the idea that children are valuable because they are important to adults. We do not feel the need to go beyond that and ask 'What is it about the child herself that means he has personal value?'.

That matters, because without a persuasive answer to that question, the value of children is subjective. It is contingent on the way that adults feel about children at the time. If, for some reason, adults chose to stop valuing children, then, in the absence of an explanation for inherent personal value, we would have to conclude

R. Hain, *Childness and the Myth of the Unfinished Human*,
https://doi.org/10.1007/978-3-032-12111-0_2

that children no longer matter. After all, it was only 2000 years ago that adults were able to overcome their protective instincts to a point where society permitted—even expected—parents to leave an unwanted child outside to die or to be eaten by wild animals. It was a mere two millennia ago that most human societies unhesitatingly allowed adults to choose to despatch a new baby who was malformed, unaffordable, or inconveniently female.

Our extraterrestrial visitor might observe that in the intervening period human society has distinctly cooled on the idea that parents should be able to decide arbitrarily what happens to their child. But she would also have to concede that traces of the same patriarchal approach have persisted well into the twentieth and twenty-first centuries. UK law, for example, still considers the deliberate killing of an infant to be less culpable than the deliberate killing of an adult. In 1922, infanticide by a mother was introduced as a form of homicide separable from murder.[1] Its primary purpose was to protect vulnerable women, but its effect is also to codify in law the idea that the life of an infant is less valuable than that of an adult.[2] The fact that, at the time of writing, society has permitted the Act to remain on the statute books is evidence that, while individual adults instinctively value individual children highly, the conglomeration of adults that we usually mean by the term 'society' (at least in the UK) is rather more ambivalent about the value of children in general, and is even willing to enshrine that differential evaluation in law.

The tendency for human society to reference the value of a child to that of adults is perhaps most clearly seen when there are difficult medical decisions to be made. In 1980, English paediatrician Dr. Leonard Arthur was charged with the murder of a newborn baby with Down's syndrome. The baby's parents said that they did not want the child because of his disability. The child was accordingly given no fluids or nutrition and died 3 days later. Writing in the *Journal of Medical Ethics* soon after the trial, barrister Diana Brahams notes that Dr. Arthur's medical record at the

---

[1] 'Where a woman by any wilful act or omission causes the death of her child being a child under the age of 12 months, but at the time of the act or omission the balance of her mind was disturbed by reason of her not having fully recovered from the effect of giving birth to the child or by reason of the effect of lactation consequent upon the birth of the child, then, if the circumstances were such that but for this Act the offence would have amounted to murder or manslaughter, she shall be guilty of felony, to wit of infanticide, and may for such offence be dealt with and punished as if she had been guilty of the offence of manslaughter of the child'. Infanticide Act 1938, Section 1(1), available at https://www.legislation.gov.uk/ukpga/Geo6/1-2/36/section/1

[2] '… in allowing a mother who kills her infant to be charged with the offence of infanticide, a lower value is placed incontrovertibly on the life of an infant under 12 months'. Helen Howard, 'The offence/defence of infanticide: A view from two perspectives', *The Journal of Criminal Law,* 82/6 (2018), 470–81. In any case, Howard points out, the Act is unnecessary, since impaired judgement as a result of psychosis occurs in men as well as women and is already a defence in law. Other experts in medical law share Howard's scepticism about the Act's utility, although more often their concern for the injustice it inflicts on the adult perpetrator rather than on the child victim (see, for example, S. H. Friedman, J. Cavney, and P. J. Resnick, 'Mothers who kill: evolutionary underpinnings and infanticide law', *Behav Sci Law,* 30/5 (Sep–Oct 2012), 585–97.: '… infanticide legislation is at best unnecessary and at worst misapplied, in that it exculpates criminal intent and fails to serve those for whom an infanticide defense might otherwise have been intended').

time shows he considered their preferences to be sufficient for deciding whether or not to intervene medically so that the child should live.[3] He was not alone; in considering that whether a child should live or die should depend on the willingness of parents to care for her, Dr. Arthur was articulating a view that most doctors of the day shared: 'A large number of eminent and respected doctors and specialists went into the witness box to testify on Dr. Arthur's behalf; he himself offered no evidence. From these many testimonies, it seemed clear that Dr. Arthur's treatment had fallen within the current accepted norms of medical practice.'[4] My point here is not to suggest that Dr. Arthur acted wrongly, but to draw attention to the reasons he gave for the actions that he took. He could have justified his decision on the grounds of compassion for the child.[5] Instead, he chose to appeal to parents' preferences in the matter, appearing to believe, as the ancient Romans and Greeks did that, even after a child has been born, parents can decide whether or not to take on the task of caring for her.

Child B was 10 years old when in 1996 she developed a rare form of leukaemia that recurred despite bone marrow transplant.[6] Bone marrow transplant is an extremely unpleasant procedure, and a second transplant will very rarely work where the first has failed; if a first transplant has not eradicated leukaemia, then the chance for cure (at least in 1996) is usually effectively zero.[7] Child B's father nevertheless insisted that a second transplant should be undertaken. When asked why, he replied that for his own peace of mind he needed to feel he had done everything he could to keep her alive. There was, in his view, no level of harm to his daughter

---

[3] 'Dr. Arthur made a note: "Parents do not wish it to survive. Nursing care only". He made out a prescription for DF118, a morphine-type drug, comprising dihydrocodeine. The drug was to be given orally, not more than four-hourly, in 5 milligram doses, to alleviate the baby's distress as and when it arose'. Diana Brahams and Malcolm Brahams, 'The Arthur Case: A Proposal for Legislation', *Journal of Medical Ethics,* 9/1 (1983), 12–15.

[4] Ibid. Sir Douglas Black, then president of the Royal College of Physicians, was one: 'I say that it is ethical, in the case of a child suffering from Down, and with a parental wish that it should not survive, to terminate life providing other considerations are taken into account such as the status and ability of the parents to cope ...' Black's use of the impersonal pronoun 'it' in referring to the baby suggests that he considered that the moral status of the child herself was negligible when compared with the interests of her parents. Dr. Arthur was ultimately acquitted following evidence that the child died as a result of complications of Down's syndrome rather than from opioid poisoning or dehydration.

[5] His actions would, in my view, have been defensible on those grounds. This particular child with Down's syndrome was severely affected and already suffering from a significant chest infection at the time the order was made. It is unlikely he could have survived more than a few days whatever interventions had been introduced. In that context, giving fluids to the child, which would have worsened many of his symptoms and demanded frequent needles, risked imposing a burden on the child that would have been hard to justify for a compassionate doctor (of whom, by common consent, Leonard was one).

[6] David Price, 'Lessons for health care rationing from the case of child B', *BMJ,* 312/7024 (1996–01–20 00:00:001996), 167–69.

[7] There are some exceptions to this, for example if the reason it fails is because the marrow (a blood-like liquid infused through a vein) does not reach its destination in the bones and so does not get a chance to work. Those cases are usually clear; Child B was not one of them.

so great that it was not justified by that benefit. It is not an unusual way of thinking among grieving parents; I myself have heard a mother say chillingly of her dying son, "I don't care how much he suffers as long as he remains alive".

These are parents who are going through the agony of losing their child. Under such circumstances, any compassionate observer would understand that the pain of an adult's grief would be overwhelming and might easily obscure all other considerations, even to the point of allowing their child to suffer unnecessarily. What is significant to the discussion in this book, however, is the response that such cases elicit from other adults in society; people who do not know the child in question and whose observations we can assume are largely disinterested. There have been recent high-profile cases in which parents have sought to make medical decisions over a dying child that the healthcare teams caring for the child believed would result in harm. Society's willingness to suborn the needs of the child to the preferences of the adult is perfectly illustrated by one anonymous social media contributor, who probably speaks for many when he or she says:

> No matter how skilled the doctors, this was NOT their decision to make, they should have recommended a course of action, of course, but NEVER ever should they have felt they had the right to impose their wishes over those of the parents.[8]

The contributor apparently believes that, in judging whether or not it is right to carry out a medical intervention in a child, the key moral question concerns the identity of the person who makes the decision. To put it another way, the contributor is suggesting emphatically that a decision over a child always, and only, becomes morally correct when it is taken by the adult parents who are caring for the child. It is a way of evaluating children that our predecessors in ancient Greece and Rome would have understood, and with which they would have identified.[9]

2.1 Intuition Is Not Enough

For most adults, the question of a child's value feels as though it has already been answered on some deep and intuitive level. Generations of adults have accorded children personal value without worrying excessively about whether or not they could account rationally for it. Such intuitions are not necessarily in tension with

---

[8] Anonymous comment on social media in relation to Charlie Gard case.

[9] No one who has cared for a family faced with losing a child would suggest, of course, that parents' preferences should be set aside or ignored. Parents usually believe they are acting for the best, and common humanity demands that doctors care for parents as well as for the child. More importantly from the point of view of informing medical decisions, parents are often best placed to provide the medical team with expert advice about what their child experiences; knowledge that is essential in making the best decision for a child. The point here, though, is that parents' preferences in the matter are not enough on their own. Contrary to what the social media contributor seemed to believe, a decision over a child does not become morally right simply because it is made by a child's parents.

what reason dictates. It seems likely that some of the ways humans instinctively think about and behave towards one another reflect 'goods' which humans might have in common with one another, and so might be said to offer a quasi-objective basis for establishing right moral behaviour. There may even be scientific explanations for them. Since genes are likely to be conserved to the extent that they increase the probability of the infant's survival into adulthood, for example, we might expect that adults would be biologically drawn to valuing children. Geneticist Richard Dawkins comments that: 'The evolutionary advantage of parental care is so obvious that ... It has been understood ever since Darwin'.[10]

But the fact that adults often *do* intuitively value children does not, of itself, constitute a demonstration that they *ought* to do so. The human intuition to care for children does not of itself provide a sufficient explanation of a child's value and, in deciding how adults should behave towards children, it would be dangerous to rely on such intuitions alone.[11] If the value of a child is contingent on the intuitions of parents, it is a volatile and fluctuating measure and the child herself is accordingly vulnerable. I have already alluded to situations in which, faced with the pain of losing a dying child, the instincts of caring parents have led them to make an evaluation of the child that is morally questionable. And we have seen that there have been times in history when society as a whole has been intuitively comfortable with actions which, in the twenty-first century, most people find intuitively repugnant. On their own, adult intuitions are an unreliable basis for an account of the child's value.

To remain persuasive in the face of society's changing perspectives on children, an account of their inherent personal value needs to appeal to some rationally defensible standard. In the past, such rational explanations were often rooted in a theological anthropology. For many, the final, ultimately ineffable, conclusion of moral debate about human value is represented by the idea that all humans, including children, have some inherent value because we all bear the image of God. At the end of the day, went the argument, humans have value because we are created by God, and God says each of us is valuable. The argument is perfectly rational, but the theist axiom on which it is based is inherently unprovable and is greeted with increasing scepticism in contemporary medical ethics. Furthermore, many bioethicists in the later twentieth and early twenty-first centuries worry that such explanations inevitably lead to the idea that all human life, and only human life, must be

---

[10] Richard Dawkins, *The Selfish Gene* (Oxford, New York: Oxford University Press, 2006), p. 108.

[11] It would be dangerous to conclude, for example, that any instinctive moral behaviour that evolution has preserved must, by the same token, be ethically right. Evolution is entirely impersonal and dispassionate and its 'concern' with human flourishing is restricted to what will ensure an individual human survives long enough for genes to be passed on through generations. As molecular biologist and moral theologian Neil Messer notes: '...all that modern biology can say is that "what all [living] things seek after" is survival and reproductive success. Biology *qua* biology gives no grounds for equating these ends with the good, in any morally informative sense, or for concluding that they are proper ends. They may be, but biology cannot tell us that they are'. Neil Messer, *Respecting life: theology and bioethics* (London: SCM Press, 2011), pp. 173–74.

preserved for as long as possible and at all costs. Reasoning about human value, some suggest, must start with a firm and explicit rejection of metaphysical ideas.[12]

2.2 Adult-Normativity and the Idea of Childness

Instinct, then, is an unreliable witness to value, and metaphysical explanations for it have lost their philosophical traction. We are left having to find an explanation for value in the infant and child that does not rely on either.

That is complicated by the plethora of different accounts of what criteria a being would have to meet in order to qualify for full personal value, and that the various accounts tend to represent a way of thinking that makes it difficult to approach the question rationally. The idea that the boundaries of personhood are simply coterminous with membership of the species *Homo sapiens* no longer seems sustainable. The idea that the moral agent should concern herself with the interests of any human being, but need not attend at all to those of non-human individuals, seems to transgress a principle of compassion as well as reason. But, if we abandon that unambiguous criterion, we are left having to decide what it is about humans that makes them, on the whole, more able than non-human animals to benefit from or be harmed by the action a moral agent might choose to take. There have been many such accounts of personal value, most of which unfortunately connect personal value with capacities that normal adults have, but that normal infants and children do not. The attributes of rationality and a capacity for exercising autonomy are, for example, normal in many adults, though perhaps rarely in an ideal form. But the same attributes would be distinctly *abnormal* if they were found in an infant or child. If we think of the ideal human being as someone with the capacity for self-rule, for example—someone who is able to reason perfectly logically, and in the actions she decides to take is able to be uninfluenced by others—then we are already thinking of an adult. That matters, because if we conclude that the way children think confers less personal value than the way adults think, then the lesser value of a child, compared with that of an adult, is assured by the child's very normality. There is a danger that we systematically undervalue the way one large group of entirely normal humans think.

---

[12]There is a risk that, along with the bathwater of dogmatism, a rejection of theological ethics throws out the substantial babies of teleology and moral realism. In dismissing the idea that human value is given by God, it can be tempting to go further and conclude that 'right' and 'wrong' simply express personal preferences for some actions over others, and have no foundation in objective truth at all. In this book, however, I will take as a starting point that ethics does have a purpose and, without conceding the consequentialist idea that only the outcome of moral action matters morally, I will assume that the ultimate object of ethically right behaviour is in some way to improve the quality of others' existence. In this book on (human) medical ethics I will focus only on the obligation of human beings to other human beings, although I fully acknowledge a broader responsibility on the part of humans to concern themselves with the well-being of members of other species.

Before examining the question of personal value in the infant or child, therefore, we have consciously to set aside any prior assumption that the way adults understand and appreciate the world is inherently the only normal way for humans to understand and appreciate the world, or even that it is the *ideal* way for all humans to understand and appreciate the world. I will describe that sort of reasoning as 'adult-normative'. If the problem facing those who wish to develop a rational account of personal value is one of normativity, then once we have decided that one way of thinking is 'more normal' or 'more nearly ideal' than others, we have already presumed the inferiority of any other way of thinking. The presumption becomes difficult to test, because it represents not only one of the comparators but also the standard against which the comparison is being made. An age-neutral approach to medical ethics necessitates rejecting any prior assumption that the cognitive characteristics and capacities that are normative for infants are inferior to those that are normative for adults.

I am going to use the term 'childness' to mean the essence of being an infant; everything that is true about an infant that does not characterise the adult and is not represented by the physicality of her material body. It is the essence ('being') of existing as a child insofar as that is different from the essence of being an adult. Childness needs to be carefully distinguished from the more familiar and related concepts 'child', 'child-like', 'childish', 'childhood' and childness. *Child* is clearly a noun describing a human who has not been alive long enough to qualify for the legal status of adult. *Child-like* and *childish* too are largely uncontentious; adjectives that connote characteristics usually associated with children but attaching to something else. They are often used to describe the behaviour of an adult. The difference between the two terms, perhaps, is that *childish* is usually pejorative while *child-like* is often used approvingly. A man with child-like qualities might be attractive, but a man who behaves childishly is merely foolish.

As Archard remarked earlier, the literal meaning of *childhood* simply denotes a period of time; an era or epoch during which a person is a child. But it is also sometimes used in a more analogical sense. When we talk of an abuser robbing someone of his or her childhood, we do not mean that their victim literally skipped the era before adulthood; we are referring to a way of existing—by implication a pleasant and fulfilling way—that is no longer open to them because the ways in which they interact with the world have been irrevocably changed. That second, analogical use of childhood begins to get close to what I mean by 'childness'. I am using childness to refer to ways of sensing and interacting with the world that characterise normal children, especially if those ways would be seen as abnormal if they were demonstrated by an adult. Importantly, the term childness is not monolithic but encompasses myriad ways of appreciating reality, just as adultness does. Since the way we sense and interact with the world depends on certain cognitive capacities, childness also implies that those capacities are present. Adultness, too, refers to ways of sensing and interacting with the world that characterise normal adults but would be seen as abnormal if they were demonstrated by a child. Again, adultness implies that the necessary capacities are present.

One reason it is important to distinguish childness carefully from those other, related, terms is that such a distinction acknowledges a gradual transition between the state of being a child and that of being an adult. An individual person cannot (other than by analogy) simultaneously be both in the era or epoch of childhood and of adulthood. He can, however, demonstrate some ways of appreciating the world that are characteristic of adults at the same time as demonstrating others that are more characteristic of children. An individual cannot at any one time be both a child and an adult, but he can certainly appreciate the world in some ways that are like an adult and others that are like a child. While the terms 'childness' and 'adultness' themselves are antithetical, in other words, at a given age someone can demonstrate both; in the same way, perhaps, that a ball can be simultaneously both black and white without having to be uniformly grey. Children themselves provide the obvious example here. Most children are hybrids who demonstrate both childness and adultness. The proportions vary from child to child. They may even fluctuate from time to time in the same child; someone who has acquired a degree of independence will often 'regress' if he becomes unwell and temporarily engage with the world as though he were more dependent. Generally, however, the usual pattern is that as the epoch of childhood progresses the individual gradually exchanges childness for adultness.

That draws attention to the newborn infant as an important exception to the general rule that children are hybrids who demonstrate both adultness and childness. Since she has not yet acquired the characteristics of adultness, the newborn child can be thought of as a child who demonstrates only childness. Much of what we now know about the cognition that characterises childness is the result of studies in the infant. At the same time, as we shall see later, because it is the infant who best exemplifies childness it is also the infant who is at greatest risk from an approach to ethics that disproportionately privileges adultness.

2.3 Summary

There is no doubt at all that individual adults care a great deal about individual children, especially, but by no means only, when those children are their own offspring. At the same time, society as a whole broadly tolerates valuing children less than adults and is happy to put the needs of adults ahead of those of children. That tolerance is reflected in medical decisions, particularly those at the end of life, when medical teams will typically allow the interests of a child to be weighed against, and sometimes even outweighed by, the preferences of her parents.

For many adults, the drive to care for an infant or child is not a conclusion reached by moral reasoning but a matter of intuition, which the current culture takes for granted. In the twenty-first century, bioethicists should not rely on such a volatile and changeable basis for evaluating children because cultural mores can easily change. Religious teaching has historically asserted the value of infants and children but, increasingly, societies no longer consider religious teaching to be a primary source of ethical guidance. We need instead to develop an account that is rationally defensible and consistent with what is empirically known about the infant and child.

Most accounts of personal value take as their starting point that the ideal way human is a normal adult, and that the ideal way for humans to appreciate and experience the world around them is in the way that a normal adult would do so. But in considering the personal value of infants and children, that prejudges the issue at hand. Instead, it is important to set aside such adult-normativity and to start (to misquote utilitarian bioethicist Peter Singer in his rejection of speciesism) with a conscious disavowal of any assumption that adults have, merely because they are adults, any distinctive worth or inherent value that puts them above younger people.[13]

Bibliography

Brahams D, Brahams M. The Arthur case: a proposal for legislation. J Med Ethics. 1983;9(1):12–5.
Dawkins R. The selfish gene. Oxford, New York: Oxford University Press; 2006.
Friedman SH, Cavney J, Resnick PJ. Mothers who kill: evolutionary underpinnings and infanticide law. Behav Sci Law. 2012;30(5):585–97.
Howard H. The offence/defence of infanticide: a view from two perspectives. J Crim Law. 2018;82(6):470–81.
Messer N. Respecting life: theology and bioethics. London: SCM Press; 2011.
Price D. Lessons for health care rationing from the case of child B. BMJ. 1996;312(7024):167–9.
Singer P. Practical ethics. New York: Cambridge University Press; 2011.

---

[13] Misquoted from Peter Singer, *Practical Ethics* (New York: Cambridge University Press, 2011), p. ix.. Singer's target is speciesism: '… it could be said that if there is any single aspect of this book that distinguishes it from other approaches to [bioethics], it is the fact that these topics are approached with a conscious disavowal of any assumption that all members of our own species have, merely because they are members of our species, any distinctive worth or inherent value that puts them above members of other species'.

Chapter 3
Childness and the Myth of the Incomplete Person

3.1 Accounting for Value

The idea that the ideal human is an adult is deeply engrained in the psyche of the human race. That is for very understandable reasons. Until recently, human society—including its philosophers—had very little to go on when it came to trying to explain a child's inherent value. Philosophy has often sought to explain inherent value on certain cognitive characteristics that an individual might possess, but those characteristics and capacities are difficult to know in an infant or child. The usual way for humans to access the experiences and thoughts of other humans is through speech, and, on the whole, children cannot talk; at least, not as well as adults do. The child is often defined precisely by her restricted ability to verbalise what she is thinking and the original meaning of the word 'infant' is simply 'one who is not yet able to speak'.[1] Until the last few decades of human history, philosophers have had no way of knowing what was going on inside the head or heart of the infant and child. In trying to explain their value, philosophers have found themselves trying to make bricks without straw.

The capacities that characterise adults, on the other hand, are qualities philosophers can understand. Not only can they draw on their own experience of and engagement with the world, but as adults themselves they can, to a certain extent, legitimately draw inferences about the way other adults do so. It seems reasonable for adults to assume that other adults have important capacities and qualities in common with themselves. If needed, philosophers are in a position to talk to other adults and find out something of what their experience of the world actually is. It is not surprising that philosophers have taken the qualities of the normal adult to be normative for all humans.

---

[1] From its Latin root *in-* ('not') and -fant from *fari* ('speaking').

R. Hain, *Childness and the Myth of the Unfinished Human*,
https://doi.org/10.1007/978-3-032-12111-0_3

The adult-normative lens through which philosophers have considered value has, however, made it difficult to say what value would look like in humans who are not adults. In the absence of a coherent and specific anthropology of the child, moral philosophy has often turned for its account of a child's value to something philosophers are much more comfortable with—the value of adults. It has found itself measuring the value of the normal child by reference to the normal adult. Broadly speaking, that has taken three forms: children are sometimes valued as the *possession* of adults, sometimes as a *prelude* to being an adult (a sort of 'trainee' adult) and sometimes as a *potential* adult. 'Possession' expresses the idea that the defining characteristic of a child is that he belongs to adults, especially his parents. According to that idea, it might not be necessary for the moral agent to disentangle the interests of the child from those of the parent. In its most extreme interpretation, a child cannot have interests that are different from those of her parents. 'Prelude' represents the value of a child in the present moment as an expression of how far her training for being an adult has progressed; the extent to which she already resembles an adult. The chronological period of childhood, on that view, is valued primarily as a period of apprenticeship which, someday, will culminate in qualification as an individual with full personal value. In this moment, the infant or child already has some value—but only to the extent that she already possesses the capacities that characterise the ideal adult.

'Potential' is usually taken to be the idea that a child is valuable now because, in the normal course of events, he will become an adult in the future. The argument goes along the lines that: 'Despite the fact that he lacks the qualities of adultness in the present moment, you should treat this child well now because one day he will acquire them'.

3.1.1 The Value of an Adult's Possession

The concept of possession expresses a relationship in which the moral agent need not concern herself with the interests of the object of her actions at all, because there are no interests to consider. A possession is a possession precisely because it has no interests of its own. The 'interests' of a possession are simply those of the possessor. A pencil cannot have any interests; when it comes to deciding on moral action in respect of a pencil, the only interests in contention are those of the person who owns it and wants to use it to write or draw. When an agent considers a moral action that will affect another normal human being, in contrast, he is expected to concern herself with the interests of that other person. Kant's formulation of that principle in 1785 is perhaps the best known: 'So act as to treat humanity, whether in thine own person or in that of any other, in every case as an end withal, never as means only'.[2]

---

[2] Immanuel Kant and Thomas Kingsmill Abbott, *Fundamental Principles of the Metaphysics of Morals* (Mineola, NY: Dover Publications, 2005).

Since the distinction between an agent's obligations to a possessed object and her obligations to another person is clear, it seems that the agent need be in no doubt about whether or not she should concern herself with the interests of either. Unfortunately, in everyday moral reasoning, there is a complication introduced by pronouns. We use the same phrase to refer to 'her pencil' and 'her mother', but we mean two quite different things. The first denotes a sense in which the moral agent need not concern himself or herself with anything other than the way in which an object will serve its owner's interests. The object exists only as a means to its owner's end; it has no end in itself. The same possessive pronoun has quite different implications, however, when it attaches to another person. There, the sense conveyed by the possessive pronoun is often that the moral agent should be *particularly* concerned about the person's own interests. A daughter is typically expected to give more weight to the interests of 'her mother', for example, than to 'a mother'. Caring for another person relies on the idea that someone else's interests can be different from your own, an idea that is specifically precluded by concepts of ownership in its purest form. Possession and care are easily conflated or confused, but in reality they are diametrically opposed when applied to beings capable of having interests.

That ambiguity is important when it comes to evaluating children, because children are definitionally part of a family group. Except in legal matters, a child is rarely 'the child'; she is always 'her', 'his', 'their' or 'my' child. It is easy to confuse the intuitive idea that parents should *care for* their child with the idea that parents might in some way be said to *possess* their child. The strongest possible illustration of parental care is, indeed, for parents to act in their child's interests when to do so means acting against their own. That is very different from the idea of the child as a possession, which, taken to extreme, might lead parents to consider that they have no need to concern themselves with the interests of the child at all.

When it comes to valuing children as possessed objects, humanity has form. Societies in the ancient world evaluated newborn babies as possessions in that latter sense; that is, they were belongings in the same way that a pencil is a belonging. The ancient world accorded parents—or at least fathers—an absolute right to decide whether or not to bring up their newborn baby.[3] That extended naturally to the idea that parents could choose to kill their baby if it served their own interests, just as they would dispose of a stylus if it became broken or if they no longer wanted or needed it.[4] While there were regions even then where infanticide was illegal, they

---

[3] '… at its birth the Greek child was so completely in its father's power that it rested with him whether or not the child should be admitted into the family. He openly signified his intention to do so during a ceremony, the *amphidromia*, which took place usually during the first week after the child's birth, at which point the child was named before the assembled members of the family and proclaimed to be a legitimate offspring. However the father had no duty to take this step'. Richard Harrow Feen, 'Abortion and Exposure in Ancient Greece', in William B. Bondeson et al. (eds.), *Abortion and the status of the fetus* (Updated reprint with corrections. Edn.; Lancaster: D. Reidel, 1983), p. 287.

[4] Aristotle appears wholeheartedly to have endorsed the practice of infanticide at parents' request, suggesting that there are circumstances under which disposing of an infant is not only permissible but morally mandatory: 'As to exposing or rearing the children born, let there be a law that no

were rare exceptions and in the ancient world most parents faced with an unwanted child would have taken the option of infanticide for granted.[5]

That casual acceptance that a parent had rights of possession over his children needs to be seen in the context of a society in which poverty was common, and the means of contraception primitive and unreliable. It was a culture in which the value of an infant's life was seen to be contingent, not on anything about the infant herself (still less the idea that the infant might have interests of her own that were relevant), but on extraneous factors such as whether or not a family's financial situation could stand the burden of another mouth to feed.[6] In these days of relative wealth and better access to contraception, most modern legislatures do not accord parents a right to dispose of unwanted children after birth. The idea that children might be possessions of adults, however, persisted for many hundreds of years after infanticide

---

deformed child shall be reared; but on the ground of number of children, if the regular customs hinder any of those born being exposed, there must be a limit fixed to the procreation of offspring, and if any people have a child as a result of intercourse in contravention of these regulations, abortion must be practised on it before it has developed sensation and life; for the line between lawful and unlawful abortion will be marked by the fact of having sensation and being alive'. Aristotle, *Politics*, trans. H. Rackham (Loeb classical library; Cambridge, MA: Harvard University Press, 1932), pp. 623–24. Aristotle does not commit himself as to at what point the human acquires a rational soul, and his positions on abortion and infanticide seem, on the face of it, to indicate contradictory ideas. He asserts uncompromisingly that there are some circumstances under which infanticide should certainly be carried out, but also expresses a view that the foetus represents an individual human life from 40 days after conception. Matthew Lu (M. Lu, 'Aristotle on abortion and infanticide', *International Philosophical Quarterly,* 53/1 (2013), 47–62 p. 50.) observes that Aristotle's comments restrict abortion only in places where there is already a societal rule prohibiting infanticide and represent a precautionary principle. The society in which Aristotle lived did not have our benefit of empirical knowledge regarding infant awareness, and he may have believed that even the infant lacked sensation and life. Aristotle recommends a 40-day limit, not because he is sure that reason has entered the foetus at that time but because, on the basis of what was known at the time, he believes himself on safe ground in assuming that before that point it has not done so. Rather than callously permitting society to deny the status of person to some humans, Aristotle might instead be compassionately arguing that there are circumstances under which society should give the status of person even to human infants, whom he believed at the time to lack the essence of personhood. Aristotle's apparently casual acceptance of infanticide would then be quite consistent with his carefully considered restrictions on abortion.

[5] Laila Williamson, 'Infanticide: an anthropological analysis', in Marvin Kohl (ed.), *Infanticide and the Value of Life* (New York: Prometheus Books, 1978), pp. 61–75.

[6] Seneca considers that disposing of imperfect infants should be a matter of reason: 'Unnatural progeny we destroy, we drown even children who at birth are weakly and abnormal. Yet it is not anger, but reason that separates the harmful from the sound'. L. Annaeus Seneca, *De Ira Liber 1. Ch. 15, sect 2.* (English translation quoted in John Wyatt, *Matters of life & death: human dilemmas in the light of Christian faith* (Nottingham: Inter-Varsity Press, 2009), p. 137.). An infant was particularly likely to be considered optional if she had had the misfortune to be born a girl. A private letter from the first century from Hilarion in Alexandria to his wife Alis is blunt on this point: 'Above all, if you bear a child and it is male, let it be; if it is female, expose it'. Hilarion, *Oxyrhincus Papyrus 4.744.*

became illegal across the Roman Empire. Thomas Hobbes, for example, wanted to argue that children are possessions of their parents, although in order to make his explanation work, he had to posit a somewhat implausible theory in which adults are invited to suppose that an infant has consented to a contractual agreement in which he accepts care at her parents' hands in return for her uncritical obedience.[7] Even in the twentieth century, bioethicist Tristram Engelhardt Jr. was still arguing that there is a defensible sense in which parents can be said to possess their offspring. Parents own a very young child, he suggests, because they have created her.[8] They also own older children and adolescents, who, ' … insofar as they remain unemancipated and fail to go out and support themselves on their own, by remaining in their parents' hands are in part owned (or, to recall the ancient Roman usage, they remain *in manu* or in parental *potestas*)'. His blunt conclusion is that young people who do not earn for themselves have, in effect, implicitly agreed to become possessions in exchange for being supported by their parents.

Most parents do not, perhaps, see the value of their child in quite the starkly contractarian terms that Hobbes or Engelhardt indicate. Nevertheless, there is evidence that the notion that parents have proprietary authority over their children persists even today. In the UK, the last decade has seen a series of cases in which a child's parents have sought to insist that doctors perform invasive interventions that were likely to be harmful to the child in some objective way and which at the same time offered little or no meaningful chance of benefit. The moral reasoning in these cases was complex and not always clear, but most referred inter alia to the idea that the child was, in some sense, her parents' child. Indeed, for many, the fact that the child was *their* child was enough to give parents an authority so great that its power should defeat even the authority of the doctors' expertise when it came to establishing the child's own interests. Ultimately in those cases it was the Courts who made the decision, and it was on the basis of what, on balance, would be best for the child. But while the cases were in the public eye, it became clear that many observers agreed that the child's parents should have the final say simply because they were the child's parents. Even where claims were less strident, many were ultimately proprietary. In his 2018 commentary on one such case, for example, bioethicist Giles

---

[7] Peter. O. King, 'Thomas Hobbes's Children', in Susan M. Turner and Gareth B. Matthews (eds.), *The philosopher's child: critical perspectives in the Western tradition* (Rochester, N.Y.; Woodbridge: University of Rochester Press, 1998), ibid. While it seems stretching credibility to suggest infants have consented to a contractual agreement, it is the nature of infants to rely on and to trust others. As we shall see later, there might therefore be an element of truth in this idea.

[8] 'One also owns what one produces. One might think here of both animals and young children. Insofar as they are the products of ingenuity or energies of persons, they can be possessions'. Engelhardt is uncomfortable with that position and almost immediately seeks to retreat from it: 'There are, however, special obligations to animals by virtue of the morality of beneficence that do not exist with regard to things. Such considerations, as well as the fact that young children will become persons, limit the extent to which parents have ownership rights over their young children'. H.T. Engelhardt, *The Foundations of Bioethics* (Oxford University Press, 1996), p. 156.

Birchley suggests that parents have what he calls 'intrinsic rights' over their child. Those rights, he suggests, do not express a responsibility to ensure the child's welfare is optimised. Rather, they are rights of possession. Referencing Locke's 'labour' explanation of ownership, Birchley explains such ownership on the basis of a certain sort of biological similarity between parent and child: 'Exploring the basis of such rights, I suggest that the strongest philosophical argument [for parental responsibility] is that Charlie was a non-person and genetically his parents' property'.[9] Birchley concedes that the idea that 'possession' authority over another person can be conferred as a result of having DNA in common with them is difficult to defend.[10] It is not clear why shared DNA might be taken to impose certain moral obligations. It would be patently ludicrous to imagine that possessing similar DNA itself is enough to explain moral relationships or ownership. That would mean that biological parents have parental privileges that adoptive ones do not, and that siblings and niblings might exercise inherent rights over one another that are denied to their spouses, and that identical twins might be said to own each other. A Lockean line of reasoning is along the lines that their shared DNA is evidence that a child's parents in some way 'created' the child, and it is their labour in doing so that gives them rights of ownership.[11] In that case, having DNA in common is morally relevant. But

---

[9] G. Birchley, 'Charlie Gard and the weight of parental rights to seek experimental treatment', *J Med Ethics,* 44/7 (Jul 2018), 448–52. Birchley offers a careful and cautious critique of such 'proprietarian accounts' and considers them to be relevant largely because the child's brain was severely damaged. Nevertheless, he accepts as a principle that there are circumstances, albeit restricted ones, under which it may be morally acceptable for parents not to concern themselves with the interests of their child; to use the child, in Kantian terms, merely as a means to parents' own end.

[10] Although such arguments continue to be made. For example, Barbara Hall, 'The Origin of Parental Rights', *Public Affairs Quarterly,* 13/1 (1999), 73–82. As recently as 2018, Birchley notes worryingly that 'Although thorough-going proprietarian arguments are rare, inclinations towards proprietarianism may be more widespread'. Birchley, 'Charlie Gard and the weight of parental rights to seek experimental treatment', p. 449.

[11] Birchley's appeal to Locke is somewhat puzzling. It is true that, in relation to objects, Locke argued that 'The labour of [a person's] body, and the work of his hands, we may say, are properly his. Whatsoever then he removes out of the state that nature hath provided, and left it in, he hath mixed his labour with, and joined to it something that is his own, and thereby makes it his property' (Locke, J. Second treatise of Government. v §27). In relation to children, however, Locke is clear that a child's relationship with her parents is defined primarily by their responsibility to concern themselves with her interests, and that any authority parents have over a child is correlative to that responsibility: 'The power, then, that parents have over their children, arises from that duty which is incumbent on them, to take care of their off-spring, during the imperfect state of childhood' (Locke, J. Second treatise of Government. vi §58). While his exclusion of children from the category of things that can be possessed might seem inconsistent with the idea that what is made can be owned, it is unequivocal and Locke's rejection of the idea that a child can be possessed is clear and emphatic. His commitment to considering children carefully in his philosophy was indeed inspired largely by his opposition to the extreme patriarchal claims of his contemporary, political theorist Robert Filmer, who affirmed an absolute right of parents over their children (Robert Filmer, *Patriarcha and Other Political Works* (first edition. Edn.; Routledge, 2017), p. 58).

only to the extent that it represents the labour that parents put into creating their offspring; it is not clear why the trivial effort of conception should be enough to confer rights of ownership over the child. Shared DNA alone cannot confer rights of ownership, nor can it, by itself, explain any significant moral obligation.

On the 'possession' view of a child's value, then, the child's value is given to her by the adult(s) whose child she is. According to the sense that we have set out, on that view the child's value expresses the degree to which the moral agent should concern herself primarily with the interests of the adults who are doing the possessing. There is a risk that the use of possessive pronouns in relation to children obscures the distinction between, on the one hand, adults' ownership of children and, on the other, their obligation to children.

3.1.2 *The Value of a Trainee Adult*

A second way in which philosophers have sought to account for inherent value in children is as 'adults-in-training'. On that account, the period of time we call childhood is conceived largely as a prolegomenon to life as an adult individual with full personal value. Its origins are perhaps in the accounts of empiricist philosophers, who understand human nature and human knowledge to result from the individual's experience of the world rather than from what can be deduced rationally. In the seventeenth century, John Locke coined the term 'tabula rasa' to describe the state of human knowledge and understanding at birth. He represents the infant as a blank tablet on which the characteristics of adulthood are gradually inscribed.[12] Those characteristics, he believes, come from the child's interaction with the world. The child accumulates knowledge over time, and there is also a gradual incrementation in the means by which knowledge is acquired, that is, rationality.[13] Locke notes that parents have obligations to their children, but he struggles to explain the basis for it.[14] He wants to argue that a child is entitled to equality with adults, but his conception of the infant as a blank slate on which, over time, knowledge is written increasingly skilfully means he has to conclude that, at any given moment, a child has to be considered less valuable than an adult.[15]

---

[12] 'Let us then suppose the mind to be, as we say, white paper, void of all characters, without any ideas:—How comes it to be furnished? ... To this I answer, in one word, from experience'. John Locke, *An Essay Concerning Human Understanding Book II: Ideas*, ed. Jonathan Bennett (2004), p. 133.

[13] D. Archard, 'John Locke's Children', in Susan M. Turner and Gareth B. Matthews (eds.), *The philosopher's child: critical perspectives in the Western tradition* (Rochester, N.Y.; Woodbridge: University of Rochester Press, 1998), p. 87.

[14] Locke, J. Second treatise of Government. vi §55. See also Ibid., pp. 93–94.

[15] 'Children, I confess, are not born in this full state of equality, though they are born to it'. Locke, J. Second treatise of Government. vi §55.

Kant, too, accords children an incremental value. He is uncomfortable with the idea that a child's interests should simply be subsumed into the interests of her parents as though they were possessions, but his focus on practical reason means he cannot easily explain why.[16] Practical reason reflects the capacity to subject oneself to the law of reason. On that view, an adult has full value as a person while the infant, understood as someone who lacks practical reason, would have no moral status and would effectively be an object.[17] At any given point in between, an individual will possess characteristics of both states. Kant considers that children have a right to be cared for, but since that right flows from the nature of family, and from marriage in particular, he struggles to explain how a child can be considered anything other than the possession of parents.[18] Kant ultimately locates the moral value of a child largely in the legal and moral right of parents to have had the child in the first place and settles uncomfortably on the idea that a child's value is somewhere between that of an adult person and an adult's possession.[19,20]

---

[16] Although Kant also holds that all human beings participate in a rational nature, even if in a given moment they are not being rational, and so should not be used as objects or 'ends in themselves': 'The ground of this principle is: Rational nature exists as end in itself. The human being necessarily represents his own existence in this way; thus to that extent it is a subjective principle of human actions. But every other rational being also represents his existence in this way as consequent on the same rational ground as is valid for me; thus it is at the same time an objective principle, from which, as a supreme practical ground, all laws of the will must be able to be derived'. Immanuel Kant, Allen W. Wood, and J. B. Schneewind, *Groundwork for the Metaphysics of Morals* (Rethinking the Western Tradition; New Haven: Yale University Press, 2002), p. 46.

[17] Although Kant stands back from that conclusion on the grounds that he considers the infant to be partly rational. Arnulf Zweig, 'Immanuel Kant's children', in Susan M. Turner and Gareth B. Matthews (eds.), *The philosopher's child: critical perspectives in the Western tradition* (Rochester, N.Y.; Woodbridge: University of Rochester Press, 1998), p. 131.

[18] Immanuel Kant, Mary Gregor, and Roger Sullivan, *Metaphysics of morals*, trans. Mary Gregor (Cambridge University Press; Cambridge: Cambridge University Press, 1996), p. 6:336. Kant's treatment of children is largely incidental to other lines of philosophical reasoning; in this instance the context is his argument that 'There are … two crimes deserving of death, with regard to which it still remains doubtful whether *legislation* is also authorized to impose the death penalty'. Dispatching an unwanted illegitimate child is one, while killing someone in a duel is the other. In both, Kant suggests, the motive for killing is honourable and the law should recognise that the legal code is at odds with other codes to which killer and killee are both subject. See also Jennifer K. Uleman, 'On Kant, Infanticide, and Finding Oneself in a State of Nature', *Zeitschrift für philosophische Forschung,* 54/2 (2000), 173–95.

[19] 'Kant's thinking about the infanticide example is probably infected also by his attitudes toward children, attitudes that are sometimes disturbingly unsentimental. Though he grants their "personhood," he does not think them as important as adults. Their deaths are less significant. Yet he does not think of a child as merely *ein Gemächsel*, an object or artifact. No being endowed with freedom (as rational or partly rational beings are) can be that'. Zweig, 'Immanuel Kant's children', in *The philosopher's child: critical perspectives in the Western tradition* p. 131.

[20] '… it is indeed in conformity with duty that the merchant should not overcharge his inexperienced customers … but rather holds a firm general price for everyone, so that a child buys just as cheaply from him as anyone else'. Kant, Wood, and Schneewind, *Groundwork for the Metaphysics of Morals*, p. 13. Kant goes on to explain carefully that, although the merchant might benefit from the reputation for fairness that such an approach would illustrate, any such benefit is incidental to the moral 'rightness' of doing so.

A prelude evaluation expresses the idea that the value of an individual child in the present moment derives from the fact that she already possesses some of the attributes that explain the value of adults.[21] At any specific point during childhood, other than its beginning, a normal child possesses some of the qualities that confer inherent value to normal adult persons and can be valued accordingly.

3.1.3 The Value of a Potential Adult

A third way of ascribing value to infants and children is on the basis of what they will one day become. While it might be difficult to ascribe inherent value to an individual in this present moment, it is clear that in the normal course of events he will one day be someone with full personal value, and a traditional argument has been that we should treat him now as though he already had that value. The inherent value of the infant or child today, on that view, is analogous to a promissory note against the value he will have when he becomes an adult.

Such an account is based on two claims. The first is the claim of teleology; that is, that the value of something is related to its purpose. That connects the value of an infant now to some goal that is inherent in infancy itself. The second is that as an organism changes over time it inevitably acquires greater value as a result of those changes, so that it is at its most valuable when they are complete. Put together, the two ideas connect the value of an infant now to the fact that he will become an adult later.

Both ideas come to us through Aristotle. The idea that value depends on purpose arose from his fundamental conviction that everything in the universe consists both in matter and form. According to that hylomorphic conception, matter is what something is made of, while form represents everything else that is true about it, including the meaning that rational beings ascribe to it. Thus, the universe 'sees' a lump of metal as a certain conformation of iron and carbon molecules without giving it any meaning; without any idea, for example, that it could be used as a knife or a paperweight. Its purpose is the meaning given to it. Only meaning-making beings are able to evaluate the qualities of sharpness or heaviness in the lump of metal, because that evaluation depends entirely on whether its purpose is to cut things or to

---

[21] Clearly there is no single point at which an individual child suddenly exchanges all the qualities of childness for those of adultness. Development is, in reality, continuous; the epoch of childhood represents a period of time over which an individual gradually loses the characteristics of childness while at the same time gradually acquiring those of adultness. A newborn infant represents the sort of child who is most different from an adult, while the adolescent child is most similar. At stages in between, the morally relevant characteristics that an individual possesses represent a mixture of those of a child and those of an adult. The proportions vary throughout childhood but represent a gradual exchange of childness for adultness. In systematising human knowledge it is often helpful to resolve such gradual changes over time into categorical distinctions (infant/child/adolescent/adult) but it is important to bear in mind that those categories are just ways of thinking; they are not ultimately part of 'the way things are'.

hold them down. Precisely the same conformation of molecules, with precisely the same physical characteristics, could be said to possess inconveniently sharp edges if its purpose is to hold things down, or to be inconveniently heavy if its purpose is to cut things. Isolated from meaning, evaluative terms like 'blunt' and 'sharp' are vacuous, saying nothing relevant at all about the value of the lump of matter they are used to describe.

Aristotle does not exclude living organisms from his hylomorphic conception of the universe. The material aspect of the organism (our physical body, for example) represents matter, while form is represented by what has been translated as 'soul'. For the purposes of this discussion, 'soul' represents everything that is true about that organism that is not represented simply by the conformation of molecules that the universe would see. It maps only broadly onto other metaphysical ideas denoted by the same term, such as theological understandings of incarnation and what happens after death. Aristotle believes that, as the matter in living organisms changes over time, so their soul (that is, everything about them that is objectively true but is not physical) also changes. The change in soul, he suggests, can be considered to occur in three stages. The most basic stage of development, the 'nutritive' soul, represents a capacity for nutrition, growth and reproduction that is possessed by all living organisms, irrespective of their level of sophistication. The second level, acquired by most non-human animals, is the 'sentient' soul. In addition to the capacities represented by a nutritive soul, organisms with a sentient soul are also capable of sensation and movement. Finally, Aristotle describes the 'rational' soul; that is, a capacity to reason, to understand and to make meaning that might include attributions of purpose.[22] Aristotle considers that it is only human beings who acquire this third level of sophistication.

Aristotle's hylomorphic anthropology is relevant to the present discussion about the value of infants and children because it links the length of time an organism has existed to an incrementation in personal value. That is often illustrated using the metaphor of an acorn.[23] Becoming an oak tree is seen to be the primary purpose

---

[22] This has sometimes led to an important confusion of ideas; namely that the cognition of infants and children is the same as that of non-human animals. Various forms of that idea persisted until the nineteenth century, most notably in the strong recapitulation theories of biologist philosopher Ernst Haeckel. Haeckel summarised his theory in the phrase 'ontogeny recapitulates phylogeny' and supported it with a series of sketches of embryos. His ideas were largely discredited when it became clear that in them Haeckel had deliberately exaggerated the similarities between species (Nick Hopwood, 'Pictures of Evolution and Charges of Fraud. Ernst Haeckel's Embryological Illustrations', *Isis,* 97/2 (2006), 260–301). We shall see later, however, that some contemporary moral philosophers continue to equate normal human cognition during infancy and childhood with the cognition of animals, presumably on the basis of Aristotle's hylomorphic anthropology.

[23] Aristotle shows that there is also a logical sense in which the way something exists in the present moment (actuality) must be more important than the idea of what it is destined to become in the future (potentiality): 'Aristotle finds that even temporally there is a sense in which actuality is prior to potentiality … A particular acorn is, of course, temporally prior to the particular oak tree that it grows into, but it is preceded in time by the actual oak tree that produced it, with which it is identical in species. The seed (potential substance) must have been preceded by an adult (actual substance). So in this sense actuality is prior even in time' (https://plato.stanford.edu/entries/aristotle-metaphysics/).

and value of an acorn; the value of the acorn must therefore always be referenced against the value of an oak tree. The value of any individual living organism must be by reference to what it is destined to become at some point in the future. Aristotle comments that, 'An animal does not become at the same time an animal or a man or a horse or any other particular animal, for the end is developed last, and the peculiar character of the species is the end of the generation in each individual'.[24] In other words, Aristotle is saying that the value of a living organism in the present moment is dependent on the organism it will eventually be. A flower is fully formed, for example, without ever acquiring a rational soul, so the fact that a flower lacks rationality is not a reason to ascribe less value to it. On Aristotelian grounds, however, a lack of rationality would be a sound reason to ascribe less value to a human being, because a human being is 'destined' to acquire both a sentient and a rational soul and is not fully formed until she does so. Since Aristotle also proposes that, during the first few years of life, an individual human being ascends through a sort of hierarchy of souls, it is clear that for Aristotle getting older is not just a matter of *chronology*, but of *maturation*; that is, progression towards a goal. As time passes, a person becomes not only older but, in some sense, gradually 'more perfect'.

On the Aristotelian view, the value of the infant must reference the infant's potential to develop into an adult, because a normal adult has acquired a rational soul, and that is the object to which human development is directed. There is a point–again, on the view Aristotle held in the fourth century BCE—at which any individual member of the species *Homo sapiens* lacks full personal value; not because he is in any way damaged, but simply because he has not yet existed for long enough to have acquired a rational soul. Although he devotes some thought to it, in the end Aristotle does not commit himself to suggesting how long that might be.[25]

Valuing the infant or child as a potential adult, then, articulates two ideas. First, the idea that increasing chronological age represents progression towards a developmental goal, so that the purpose of an infant or child is to become an adult. Second, the idea that such progression represents a change in value. On that account, the value of an infant or child in the present moment is, in effect, a sort of 'promissory

---

[24] Aristotle, *On the generation of animals*, p. II:2.

[25] That is because, on the hylomorphic view, you would need to be able to identify a sense organ for rationality in order to identify empirically the point at which an individual member of the species *Homo sapiens* becomes fully a person. Whereas Aristotle was clear that an early embryo has no sentient soul because it lacks the organs of sense, he thought there was no analogous sense organ for rationality and found himself forced to conclude that there is no empirical way of telling when an individual human being becomes a person with full personal value. It is interesting to consider what Aristotle would have made of the empirical evidence we now have regarding a newborn infant's neuroanatomy and cognitive capacities.

note' against the value she will have as an adult in the future. An argument from potential, as it is often understood in the twenty-first century, represents the value of an infant today in terms of what he is expected to become in the future. When deployed against infanticide, for example, the argument from potential is that the infant's life is valuable because, all things being equal, there is an expectation that the infant will one day become a normal adult. Those who deploy the argument from potential typically suggest that the value of the infant as a potential adult should be considered equal to the value of an actual adult.

3.2   The Argument from Potential and Its Problems

There seems little doubt that expressing the value of an infant in terms of the value of the adult she is destined to become has historically offered some protection to children, and especially infants, who might otherwise have been undervalued. Some consequentialist philosophers, however, regard the argument from potential as a moral 'sleight of hand', designed to assure human infants of a special status for which they believe there is no rational explanation. Why should an individual be allowed to borrow value today from the value of the person she might or might not become in the future, simply on the basis that she is human?[26] Writing in the 1970s, bioethicist Michael Tooley sets out the utilitarian objection to the argument from potential using a thought experiment in which he posits a chemical that, if injected into a kitten, would imbue the kitten with all the attributes of moral status enjoyed by adult humans.[27] Having received the injection, Tooley considers that the kitten would become human in all ways relevant to how it should be treated by other humans. Tooley goes on to point out that there would be nothing immoral in choosing to withhold that injection from the kitten so that it remained a non-human kitten.[28]

---

[26] Singer, *Practical Ethics*, p. 68.

[27] 'Suppose at some future time a chemical were to be discovered which when injected into the brain of a kitten would cause the kitten to develop into a cat possessing a brain of the sort possessed by humans, and consequently into a cat having all the psychological capabilities characteristic of adult humans. Such cats would be able to think, to use language, and so on. Now it would surely be morally indefensible in such a situation to ascribe a serious right to life to members of the species *Homo sapiens* without also ascribing it to cats that have undergone such a process of development: there would be no morally significant differences'. Michael Tooley, 'Abortion and Infanticide', *Philosophy & Public Affairs,* 2/1 (1972), 37–65 p. 36.

[28] '[I]t would not be seriously wrong to refrain from injecting a new-born kitten with the special chemical, and to kill it instead. The fact that one could initiate a causal process that would transform a kitten into an entity that would eventually possess properties such that anything possessing them *ipso facto* has a serious right to life does not mean that the kitten has a serious right to life even before it has been subjected to the process of injection and transformation. The possibility of transforming kittens into persons will not make it any more wrong to kill new-born kittens than it is now' (Ibid.). Helga Kuhse suggests that Tooley's argument here is inconsistent with his defence of abortion and infanticide, because those defences rely on the quality of a person's existence in

If it would not be wrong to withhold a 'humanness' injection from the cat in his thought experiment, he goes on, then on the same reasoning it would not be wrong to prevent a human infant from acquiring full moral status. Tooley holds the view that the infant's cognitive limitations, like those of a cat, mean the infant does not possess the attributes of full moral status in the here and now, and he dismisses as irrelevant the future possibility of adulthood because it does not describe any properties of the infant at the moment moral action is considered. After all, if the infant is despatched today, then the question of what she might become in the future future is emphatically and unambiguously resolved.

Writing 40 years later, Giubilini and his colleagues caricature the argument from potential along lines that are essentially the same as Tooley's, repeating his claim that, in the present moment, the infant is not a person at all but rather a 'potential' person, and that speculative ideas about what might or might not happen to her in the future are of no relevance when it comes to informing what action a moral agent should take in the present.[29] Philosopher Cecil 'Tony' Coady goes further and suggests that describing something as potential means that the object to which it attaches does not exist at all. Prepending the adjective 'potential', Coady insists, logically denies the existence of any object to which it refers, in the same way that the adjectives 'decoy' and imaginary' do. While 'a happy dog is of course a dog', he points out, '… a potential champion is not yet a champion of any sort'.[30]

The idea that an infant's value might vest in what he will become certainly puts the doctor as a moral agent in a difficult position in practice. Decisions regarding

---

the future which he has dismissed as irrelevant in his 'kitten' metaphor: 'If one accepts Tooley's argument that there is an obligation to refrain from bringing wretched people into the world, then one must also accept the reverse: an obligation exists to bring additional happy people into the world. In this case, both abortion and infanticide are wrong'. Helga Kuhse, 'Michael Tooley on possible people and promising', *Camb Q Healthc Ethics,* 2/3 (Summer 1993), 353–8.

[29] Despite the advances in understanding in developmental neuropsychology in the intervening years, Giubilini and colleagues, like Tooley, take as their starting axiom that the capacities that characterise human personhood exclude any of the capacities that characterise childness: 'It might be claimed that someone is harmed because she is prevented from becoming a person capable of appreciating her own being alive. Thus, for example, one might say that we would have been harmed if our mothers had chosen to have an abortion while they were pregnant with us or if they had killed us as soon as we were born. However, whereas you can benefit someone by bringing her into existence (if her life is worth living), it makes no sense to say that someone is harmed by being prevented from becoming an actual person. The reason is that, by virtue of our definition of the concept of "harm" in the previous section, in order for a harm to occur, it is necessary that someone is in the condition of experiencing that harm' (A. Giubilini and F. Minerva, 'After-birth abortion: why should the baby live?', *J Med Ethics,* 39/5 (May 2013), 261–3).

[30] 'We must be wary of the traps that can beset the use of adjectives like "potential". "Potential" does not function in the way many standard adjectives do. A happy dog is of course a dog, as a snappy tie is a tie, or a sad face a face. But just as a decoy duck is emphatically not a duck and an imaginary win is not a victory at all, so a potential champion is not yet a champion of any sort'. C. A. Coady, 'The common premise for uncommon conclusions', *J Med Ethics,* 39/5 (May 2013), 284–8 p. 285.

moral action over an infant need to be made in the here and now. If 'potential' expresses no more than the possibility that the child in front of her will reach adulthood, the doctor finds herself having solely on account of hypothetical value at some point in the future. That is of limited help at the moment she needs to make a decision, because the fact that *most* infants will become adults does not mean that this *particular* infant will become an adult, and it would be problematic to evaluate him today purely on the grounds that he will. The mere possibility that an individual will demonstrate adultness in 15 or 20 years' time—however great that possibility might be—is perhaps of little relevance to how the agent should treat him today when he demonstrates only childness. Furthermore, there are individuals who, it is quite certain, will never acquire the cognitive skills of adultness (for example, children who are terminally ill), or who could only acquire adultness if their circumstances were changed (for example, children living in poverty or out of reach of curative medical interventions).[31] Those are often, by the same token, children who are particularly vulnerable and whose interests in the present moment should be of especial concern to the moral agent. A narrowly probabilistic conception of potential is multiply problematic as a sole source of explanation for a child's value.

3.2.1 Potential as Nature

That probabilistic idea of potential-as-probability is not, however, the one that has shaped the argument from potential. Moral theologian Charles Camosy points out that, historically, the meaning of the term 'potential' was not restricted to something about an infant that might *become* true in the future, but rather indicated something about the infant that is *already* true in the present moment.[32] In the Christian theological terms that served to discredit infanticide in the ancient world, 'potential'

---

[31] See Charles Camosy: 'Some might argue here that Patrick's potential for gaining personal capacities is actually a fiction. No such treatment exists and thus the potential is zero. However, this is … mathematical potential (or 'probability') rather than potential of kind or nature. Such mathematical potential can be influenced by a host of factors that have no moral relevance — many of them social. Consider that an infant born with bone cancer may have a mathematical probability of becoming a person of zero given her social situation (say, she is born in the remote areas of a developing country with no technology to treat such a disease), but that means nothing for her actual moral status — in light of her natural potential for personhood. Indeed, such potential would be realized if she lived in a different social situation'. Charles Camosy, *Too Expensive to Treat?: Finitude, Tragedy, and the Neonatal ICU* (W.B. Eerdmans Publishing Company, 2010), p. 57.

[32] '… passive potential (or mere probability) adds nothing to the moral status of an entity, but the Church's 'substance' position is that any being of a rational nature—that is, a being with active potential for personal traits–counts as a person. Membership in the species Homo sapiens, though not significant in and of itself, does indicate what really matters morally about the fetus and infant: their being substances of a rational nature'. Charles Camosy, 'Engaging with Peter Singer', in John Perry (ed.), *God, the good, and utilitarianism: perspectives on Peter Singer* (Cambridge: Cambridge University Press, 2014), p. 192. Camosy suggests somewhat optimistically that this

represented an individual's nature; the unique set of ways in which each individual human both participates and does not participate in what generally enables humans to flourish.

The importance of that broader understanding of potential-as-nature is illustrated by Coady's questionable assertion that the adjective 'potential' negates the existence of the noun to which it is applied. He is wrong to suggest that 'imaginary', 'decoy' and 'potential' all have comparable effects on the object they describe, or that none of them expresses anything about the nature of the object in the present moment. It is true that a win that is imaginary has, by definition, no existence in the present moment. But that is because of the specific meaning of the adjective 'imaginary'. The effect of other adjectives would be different. A decoy duck, for example, certainly *does* exist in the present moment. Furthermore, even if the value of a decoy duck is not the same as that of a living duck, its value indisputably depends on the extent of its resemblance to an actual waterfowl of the family *Anatidae*. Calling something a 'decoy' duck firmly links its current value, not only with the existence of an actual duck, but also with the nature of one, since a decoy that lacked any resemblance to a duck would be of no value at all.

Similarly, while it is true that calling someone a 'potential' champion should not be taken to mean that her prowess is the same as that of an actual champion, as a description it is not merely speculation about her future but represents a relevant evaluative statement about her in the present moment.[33] There are people in the present moment who cannot be reasonably described as potential champions, because as a matter of fact they lack the necessary attributes. There are other people who (again, in the present moment) do have those attributes and can be so described. It is true of me that I neither speak Portuguese nor play professional tennis. I have a flair for language, however, and so it would be reasonable to describe me as a potential speaker of Portuguese. On the other hand, I have no talent whatsoever for ball games and no reasonable person who has ever seen me try would describe me as a 'potential professional tennis player'.[34] The fact that I have one potential but not the other expresses something that is true about me now (*in the present moment* I am good at languages but lack hand–eye coordination). It does not express only what might or might not become true about me later on.

---

disagreement between Singer and Christian ethics about the relevance of passive potential is 'very narrow'.

[33] Later in the same paper, Coady seems to acknowledge this when he remarks, apparently inconsistently: 'None of this is to deny, of course, that the potentiality of an entity sometimes provides a reason for according it some value or respect.' Coady, 'The common premise for uncommon conclusions', p. 285.

[34] This illustrates that the idea of potential-as-nature can express a limitation on what a being can become, as well as its extent. An infant's nature represents the limits of what she might achieve. She might well grow up to become less than her nature would have permitted (for example, if she sustained a brain injury), but even if she were not injured, she could not grow up to become *more* than her nature permitted.

A child's potential-as-nature expresses something about her now, so that a child can meaningfully be said to have potential even if there is no possibility that he will survive to adulthood.[35] If potential expresses something about what the individual is objectively like in the present moment, then even on utilitarian grounds Giubilini and Coady have not argued away entirely its moral relevance in evaluating an individual, because the concept of potential-as-nature directly connects it to how the moral agent should treat her in the here and now.

A more practical objection to the argument from potential-as-nature is that it does not provide a clear solution mechanism in medical decision-making because it introduces complexities into the connection between the nature of the patient and the action that a doctor should take. A consequentialist analysis is straightforward: a consequentialist argument for infanticide, for example, might simply be that killing an infant today would not harm her today in any meaningful sense because she lacks self-awareness or a sense of futurity. The logic is clear and presents no difficulties. An objection to infanticide from potential-as-nature takes a far more convoluted route, arguing firstly that it is wrong to kill persons, then that the reason humans are persons is that they are characterised by a distinctive capacity for reasoning that includes self-awareness and futurity, and then that, because infants are human, and humans normatively have such a rational nature, it is the infant's nature to be rational. Only then does an argument from potential finally arrive at the conclusion that it is wrong to kill infants.[36] The practical connection between someone's attributes, and the rightness of a moral action, which is so obvious and so direct in most forms of utilitarianism, is something of a 'knight's move' in arguments from potential.

---

[35] Camosy, *Too Expensive to Treat?*, p. 57.

[36] Singer's mentor and author of preference utilitarianism R. M. Hare argues on utilitarian grounds that even passive potential is enough to account for full value in the fetus: 'The potentiality of the embryo to develop into someone who can enjoy the listed benefits (let us say for short "into a grown person") is important just because, if it does, that grown person will benefit. The benefit is not to the embryo. Nor is it to the foetus [sic] or even the neonate. The preservation of embryos, foetuses and neonates is important just because if they are preserved they will turn into grown people who will benefit from existing (not indeed because bare existence in itself is a benefit, but because in normal circumstances those who exist can have other benefits like those listed)'. R. M. Hare, 'When does potentiality count? A comment on Lockwood', *Bioethics,* 2/3 (Jul 1988), 214–26 p. 216. Contrast with M. Lockwood, 'Hare on potentiality: a rejoinder', *Bioethics,* 2/4 (Oct 1988), 343–52.

3.2.2   Potential and Adult-Normativity

If 'potential' is taken to express no more than the possibility of something in the future, then Coady is right to the extent that he suggests that describing something as potential might modify its value. Even on those terms, however, it is not immediately obvious why calling something 'potential' should inevitably remove *all* its value in the present moment. Aristotle does not suggest, for example, that becoming an oak tree is an acorn's *only* purpose. Even if we decide to disregard today any value that derives from the acorn's potential to become an oak tree in the future, we are still left with the possibility that an acorn might have some value in the present moment. Acorns make good pig food, for example.[37] Similarly, if we disregard today any value the infant derives from her potential to become an adult in the future, we are still left with the possibility that he might have some value in the present moment. Unless, of course, we have already decided axiomatically that we will not ascribe value to the infant. If we agree with Coady that calling an infant a 'potential' adult removes all her value, it is not because of anything about the adjective itself, but for the adult-normative reason that we have already decided childness is less valuable than adultness.

It is as a defence against such casual devaluing of infants that the argument from potential-as-probability is typically deployed. It proposes a way in which a being can have value in the present moment despite lacking the cognitive capacities that normatively characterise adults. Such a defence does not, however, challenge an adult-normative moral anthropology because its expression of the value of a child is not in terms of childness, but of adultness. It reflects a way of valuing the infant in which her value today represents only what can be borrowed from her future self—a future self who will have acquired the inherent value that adultness can confer. Underlying this view is the assumption that maturation is inevitably linked to an increase in moral status. That perpetuates the idea that an infant's purpose is solely to exchange childness for adultness, and so restricts the value of childness to the extent to which childness can facilitate adultness.

An analogy might be if you were invited to pick as many apples as you like for free from an orchard, provided you bring along your own basket to put them in. Because you like apples, you hasten home to find a basket but find that the only one

---

[37] 'One cannot speak of the flourishing of any kind without implicitly indicating a wider order which will determine what flourishing and frustration within that kind consist of. An acorn flourishes by becoming an oak; but why should this be a more successful thing for it to become than pig's food? We have to choose between a purely anarchistic answer, based on an ultimate competition between all species, and an answer which points to the value for other beings of there being oaks and not just acorns'. Oliver O'Donovan, *Resurrection and Moral Order: an Outline for Evangelical Ethics* (second edn.; Leicester: William B. Eerdmans Pub. Co., 1994), pp. 34–35.

you have is already full of peaches. For the purpose of this illustration, there is no way of keeping peaches other than in the basket, so at this point you are faced with a decision: do you keep the peaches or throw them away so that you can fill the basket with apples instead? Fortunately, you do not like peaches as much as apples, so you empty them all out and take the now-empty basket to the orchard in order to fill it with the fruit you prefer. Your willingness to throw the peaches away represents a judgement about the relative value of apples and peaches. If you prefer apples to peaches, you might see the basket as a potential basket of apples, even if it is currently full of peaches, whereas if you value apples and peaches equally, you will see it instead as an actual container of peaches. Similarly, valuing an infant or child today primarily on the basis that one day she will be characterised by adultness, rather than on the basis that today she is characterised by childness, represents a judgement that adultness is more valuable than childness. An argument from potential-as-probability—the idea that an infant's value can be entirely expressed by the chance that she will become an adult—is problematic on age-neutral terms because it represents an adult-normative conception of personal value.

An argument from potential-as-nature is more promising, but it too cannot wholly express an infant's present value unless it is coupled with an acknowledgement of the value of childness. Camosy suggests that a claim for potential-as-nature is tantamount to a claim that '… all newly born infants have the dignity and worth of persons, [and] the good of their lives cannot be directly acted against in infanticide'.[38] He seems to be claiming that, because an argument from potential-as-nature demonstrates that the life of infants has *some* inherent value, by the same fact it demonstrates that the inherent value of the infant's life is the same as that of the adult. While his conclusion that the infant has inherent value of the infant is valid, in reaching it Camosy seems to have made too great a logical leap. He is right to suggest, *contra* many utilitarians, that potential-as-nature confers *some* value on an individual life in the present moment. But surely those are not sufficient grounds for concluding that the value of the present infant is *the same as* the value of an actual present adult, any more than, as we have seen, a potential champion is already the same as a champion. Showing that an acorn has some value because its nature is characterised by 'oakness' does not, on its own, justify concluding that its value is already that of an oak tree. Camosy must be right that potential-as-nature confers some inherent personal value. But unless it is coupled with an acknowledgement that childness and adultness are equally valuable attributes of that nature, even an argument from potential-as-nature does not rule out the possibility that, in this moment, an infant might be less valuable than an adult.

---

[38] Camosy, *Too Expensive to Treat?*, pp. 61–62.

3.3   Stacking the Odds: Adult-Normativity as Systematic Ethical Bias

The ways in which moral philosophy has sought to express human value have often been unable to account convincingly for the value of a child in her own right. While most philosophers have felt intuitively that the moral agent ought to care for children, they have often struggled to find in their moral theories an explanation for that obligation. Philosophy has found itself instead having to express the child's value by reference to the adults around her. For some theorists, a child's value is seen to be an expression of the value that is given to her by her adult owners. For others, it is an expression of the morally relevant cognitive capacities that, in the present moment, she already has in common with adults. For others again, her value is an expression of her potential to become an adult in the future.

What those accounts have in common is that they avoid having to ascribe value to childness itself. They all say, in effect, 'It is the qualities that are specifically normative for adult humans that confer personal value. In order to evaluate a child, we cannot turn to the qualities he possesses that are specifically normative for children, because those are not the qualities that confer personal value. In order to explain his value, we need to turn to some other source. Reference to adults can provide that source. The child is valuable because adults want him, or because he already demonstrates some of the qualities of adultness that *can* confer inherent value or because, in the fulness of time, he might become an adult'.

All three of those explanations for a child's value rely on the same underlying fundamental conviction that it is the capacities that characterise adults that provide the yardstick for evaluating all persons; that it is possession of the capacities that characterise adults that represents full human personhood. When the moral agent evaluates a child on the basis that he is the possession of adult, or as someone in training to become an adult, or as a potential adult, she is demonstrating adult-normative thinking. She is evaluating the infant or child by reference to qualities that are normative for an adult.

The result is that moral philosophy has failed to develop a coherent account of the value of a child that emanates from an anthropology of the child herself, one that relies on the qualities that are normative for a child.

Adult-normativity in moral philosophy introduces an important systematic bias. If children are evaluated by reference to adults, then normal children are condemned to lesser value by their very normality. If, for example, rational autonomy, a sense of futurity, or the capacity to express preferences is considered to be criteria for full personal value, then the normal child cannot be fully a person *ex hypothesi* because the normal child does not have rational autonomy, a sense of futurity, or the capacity to express preferences.

3.3.1   The Particular Vulnerability of Infants

Childness and adultness are antithetical terms because each is defined by contrast with the other. A person's change from child to adult, however, is a matter of change in form—a gradual transition from one thing into a different thing. A thing and the description of a thing are separable from each other. A ball can be black, but it can also be white.

Childness and adultness are collections of attributes, rather than monolithic or unitary features. They can, and often do, operate simultaneously; a single individual at a given point in time might appreciate and make sense of the world in some ways that represent childness and others that represent adultness.

The gradual change from child to adult nevertheless represents a progressive doffing of the characteristics of childness, at the same time as a progressive donning of characteristics of adultness. In that case, there must be a time when any given individual possesses overwhelmingly the characteristics of childness—a point in her life when the characteristics of childness predominate to such a degree that those of adultness pale into inconsequence. It seems reasonable to locate that at the time of birth. It is the newborn child who illustrates most clearly the cognitive characteristics that I have grouped together and labelled 'childness'. I have suggested that our current approach to medical ethics systematically undervalues childness. If I am right, then the extent to which a given individual is vulnerable to such undervaluing is the extent to which she demonstrates childness. Since it is the infant who demonstrates childness at its most unadulterated (so to speak), it is the infant who is most vulnerable to that systematic bias. It is the infant who finds herself in a closed logical loop, in which all the characteristics and capacities she possesses are evaluated by reference to characteristics and capacities that she is inherently excluded by virtue of her normality from ever possessing. No bioethical theory can adequately serve those whom it imprisons inside such an evaluative logical loop.

3.4   Summary

Moral philosophy has often struggled to account rationally for the inherent value of children because it has relied on accounts of personal value that derive from knowledge of adults and the way adults see the world. For most of human history, little was known, or could be discovered, about how children appreciate and experience the world, whereas the way adults do so was easily accessible. It is understandable that philosophers should have seen ethics through a lens that was 'adult-normative'; that is, based on the assumption that the ideal way for humans to appreciate and experience the world is the way that normal adults do so.

Since children are relatively different, philosophers have struggled to find a place for children in their moral theories. Where they have done so, they have often found themselves having to evaluate children by reference to adults; as possessions valued by their adult owner, for example, or as those who have acquired some, but not all, the characteristics of adults. The value of infants has been particularly difficult to explain on those terms. For the purposes of this discussion, an infant represents a human at the stage where childness predominates most markedly over adultness, and who is therefore most vulnerable to an account of bioethics that systematically undervalues childness. One philosophical 'work-around' has been the argument from potential; a way of explaining the value of an infant in the here and now by referencing it to what, in the normal way of things, he will become in the future. Historically, the argument has served to protect infants, but rationally it is not wholly persuasive. If it refers to nothing more than the probability that an infant will some-day develop the capacities that do confer full personal value, then it is not always clear in the individual case why potential should require the moral agent to consider the interests of the infant today. Furthermore, on those grounds, there are patients to whom a doctor owes no obligation because it is certain for medical reasons that they will never develop those capacities.

Abandoning adult-normative thinking makes it even more problematic to value an infant according to how likely it is that she will become an adult, because the argument from potential-as-probability is predicated on the idea that an individual gains in value as she matures. The argument becomes unsustainable in the face of an approach that disavows the presupposition that adultness is inherently more valuable than childness.

If, instead, potential is considered to represent an individual's nature—the extent and limitations of her abilities, for example—then it describes something that is already true about the infant. There is a direct connection between the present cognitive capacities of the moral patient and the obligations of the moral agent—one that does not rely on speculation about the future. An argument from potential-as-nature succeeds, even on consequentialist grounds, in attributing some inherent value to the infant in the present moment.

Those grounds alone, however, leave open the possibility that the moral agent should concern herself less with the interests of an individual during infancy than during adulthood. To avoid such systematic undervaluation of the infant, it will be necessary to evaluate the normative characteristics of infants on their own terms, and not by reference to those of adults at all. An argument from potential-as-nature can only accord the infant the same value as the adult if it is coupled with the idea that the way in which an individual participates in that nature as an infant is of the same value as the way in which he would do so as an adult. On those age-neutral terms, the value of an individual who happens to be an infant in the present moment is expressed by the extent to which he is already able to flourish as that particular infant, and not by the probability that he will one day come to resemble an ideal adult.

Bibliography

Archard D. John Locke's children. In: Turner SM, Matthews GB, editors. The philosopher's child: critical perspectives in the Western tradition. Rochester, Woodbridge: University of Rochester Press; 1998.

Aristotle. Politics, Loeb classical library; trans. Rackham H. Cambridge, MA: Harvard University Press; 1932.

Aristotle. On the generation of animals. c 350 BC.

Birchley G. Charlie Gard and the weight of parental rights to seek experimental treatment. J Med Ethics. 2018;44(7):448–52.

Camosy C. Too expensive to treat?: finitude, tragedy, and the neonatal ICU. W.B. Eerdmans Publishing Company; 2010.

Camosy C. Engaging with Peter Singer. In: Perry J, editor. God, the good, and utilitarianism: perspectives on Peter Singer. Cambridge: Cambridge University Press; 2014.

Coady CA. The common premise for uncommon conclusions. J Med Ethics. 2013;39(5):284–8.

Engelhardt HT. The foundations of bioethics. New York: Oxford University Press; 1996.

Filmer R. Patriarcha and other political works. 1st ed. Routledge; 2017.

Giubilini A, Minerva F. After-birth abortion: why should the baby live? J Med Ethics. 2013;39(5):261–3.

Hall B. The origin of parental rights. Public Aff Q. 1999;13(1):73–82.

Hare RM. When does potentiality count? A comment on Lockwood. Bioethics. 1988;2(3):214–26.

Harrow Feen R. Abortion and exposure in ancient Greece. In: Bondeson WB, et al., editors. Abortion and the status of the fetus. Updated reprint with corrections ed. Lancaster: D. Reidel; 1983.

Hilarion. Oxyrhincus Papyrus 4.744.

Hoffmaster B. The rationality and morality of dying children. Hast Cent Rep. 2011;41(6):30–42.

Hopwood N. Pictures of evolution and charges of fraud. Ernst Haeckel's embryological illustrations. Isis. 2006;97(2):260–301.

Kant I, Abbott TK. Fundamental principles of the metaphysics of morals. Mineola: Dover Publications; 2005.

Kant I, Gregor M, Sullivan R. Metaphysics of morals (trans. Gregor M). Cambridge: Cambridge University Press; 1996.

Kant I, Wood AW, Schneewind JB. Groundwork for the metaphysics of morals. Rethinking the Western tradition. New Haven: Yale University Press; 2002.

King PO. Thomas Hobbes's children. In: Turner SM, Matthews GB, editors. The philosopher's child: critical perspectives in the Western tradition. Rochester, Woodbridge: University of Rochester Press; 1998.

L. Annaeus Seneca De Ira Liber 1. Ch. 15, sect 2.

Locke J. In: Bennett J, editor. An essay concerning human understanding book II: ideas. New York: Penguin Books; 2004.

Lockwood M. Hare on potentiality: a rejoinder. Bioethics. 1988;2(4):343–52.

Lu M. Aristotle on abortion and infanticide. Int Philos Quart. 2013;53(1):47–62.

O'Donovan O. Resurrection and moral order: an outline for evangelical ethics. 2nd ed. Leicester: William B. Eerdmans Pub. Co; 1994.

Singer P. Practical ethics. New York: Cambridge University Press; 2011.

Uleman JK. On Kant, infanticide, and finding oneself in a state of nature. Z Philos Forsch. 2000;54(2):173–95.

Williamson L. Infanticide: an anthropological analysis. In: Kohl M, editor. Infanticide and the value of life. New York: Prometheus Books; 1978.

Wyatt J. Matters of life & death: human dilemmas in the light of Christian faith. Nottingham: Inter-Varsity Press; 2009.

Zweig A. Immanuel Kant's children. In: Turner SM, Matthews GB, editors. The philosopher's child: critical perspectives in the Western tradition. Rochester, Woodbridge: University of Rochester Press; 1998.

Kuhse H. Michael Tooley on possible people and promising. Camb Q Healthc Ethics. 1993;2(3):353–8.

Tooley M. Abortion and infanticide. Philos Public Aff. 1972;2(1):37–65.

Chapter 4
Adult-Normativity: An Unreliable Measure

If the problem with ethical thinking about the value of infants and children were simply that philosophers had too little to go on, it seems that in the twenty-first century it should be relatively easy to resolve. Science has revealed a great deal about the cognitive abilities of newborn infants and today we have some good evidence, both about what cognitive equipment the infant possesses and about how she uses it in practice to understand the world and herself in relation to it. Those are essentially empirical questions and, while there are still obstacles to our knowing more about them, the obstacles are practical ones, some of which may crumble as time passes. No one today can claim with any authority that childness represents no more than the absence of adult cognitive capacities. It might seem that those who have argued that the cognitive capacities of childnes are of no inherent value should now simply capitulate in the face of the evidence. Its nature is no longer an arcane mystery, and what we now know about it makes some historical claims about the infant quite implausible.

Yet many continue to argue that, when it comes to conferring personal value, the way infants appreciate their existence is of less value than that of adults. Today, there are more moral philosophers than ever who judge an infant's life to have little or no inherent value, and who defend that judgement by an appeal to the sort of thinking that the infant cannot do. That suggests the problem has not been simply that philosophers were unaware of an infant's capabilities, but that there is something else going on in their thinking that persuades them to assert that some or all of what an infant *can* do should be set aside as irrelevant.

R. Hain, *Childness and the Myth of the Unfinished Human*,
https://doi.org/10.1007/978-3-032-12111-0_4

4.1 The Child in an Adult-Normative World

While a better knowledge of what the infant can do must go some way towards help-ing moral theorists to accord childness its proper value, it is not enough on its own. Even in the face of a more precise understanding of the cognitive capabilities that characterise childness, it would remain open to the theorist to decide that those capabilities are less valuable than what characterises adultness. Correctly ascribing value to, or withholding it from, an infant demands epistemic accuracy as well as a sound knowledge of empirical data. It depends on which of the characteristics and capabilities that constitute childness the theorist considers should 'count'. In the opening chapter of this book, I quoted contemporary ethicist John Wall, who notes that: '… Across diverse societies and cultures, and throughout history and today, serious questions of human being, purposes, and responsibilities have usually been considered chiefly from the point of view of adulthood. Childhood has had to borrow its senses of meaning and humanity from those thought to embody them in some fuller, more advanced, or more important way.'[1]

The conclusions that moral philosophy has often reached about the value of childness reflect not only an imperfect knowledge of neurodevelopmental psychol-ogy, but also a judgement that the capacities of adultness somehow embody mean-ing and humanity in a 'fuller, more advanced or more important way' than those of childness. They have already reached a conclusion about what capacities and attri-butes matter to personal value and which do not. The central idea that bioethicist Peter Singer expresses in his preference utilitarian defence of infanticide, for exam-ple, is a quintessentially adult-normative. It might be reasonable, Singer concedes, for a society to choose to restrain its members from killing babies, but any such limitation should be justifiable on the grounds of the impact it would have on adults. It should not be taken to imply anything about the inherent value of the infant her-self. The moral 'rightness' of preserving an infant's life is fully explained by the suffering her death would cause to adults.[2] He is urging th   at the difference in value between childness and adultness is so great that the moral agent should con-cern herself more with the mere preferences of beings who exhibit adultness than with the life or death of those who exhibit only childness.

One way to explain Singer's overwhelming privileging of adults over children is that he has evaluated children against a yardstick that has been developed with adults in mind. Earlier, we saw that bias can be inadvertently programmed into autonomous vehicles if developers train the vehicles to think too narrowly about what a pedestrian looks like. In training the vehicle to associate the characteristics of a pedestrian too closely with those of an adult, the developers ensure that the vehicle will sometimes fail to recognise a child as a pedestrian at all. The car's resul-tant willingness to kill infants and children is a result of adult-normative thinking on the part of the car (and, indirectly, on the part of its developers).

---

[1] Wall, *Ethics in light of childhood*, p. 1.

[2] '… these restrictions should owe more to the effects of infanticide on others than to the intrinsic wrongness of killing an infant. Obviously, in most cases, to kill an infant is to inflict a terrible loss on those who love and cherish the child'. Singer, *Practical Ethics*, p. 154.

Clinical medicine provides other analogies for the danger that adult-normativity can pose to infants and children. A sphygmomanometer (blood pressure machine), for example, consists of a pressure monitor attached to an inflatable cuff that goes around a patient's arm. The cuff is positioned over an artery in the arm and inflated to a point where the pressure it exerts equals the pressure generated by the heart's pumping and transmitted through the blood running through the artery. Because the pressures are now equal, the cuff is able to compress the artery; the blood stops flowing smoothly and the sound of that turbulence can be detected by the machine or through a stethoscope. A standard sphygmomanometer cuff will give an accurate and repeatable measure of an individual adult's blood pressure.

If, however, the same blood pressure cuff is used to measure blood pressure in children, it becomes systematically unreliable, because the pressure exerted by the cuff depends not only on the actual blood pressure, but also on how big the cuff is relative to the size of the patient's arm. Used in a child, the machine will return a value. That value will be superficially plausible and might easily be taken to be a reliable observation, but in fact it will be significantly lower than the child's actual blood pressure. The reason, of course, is that the normal child is smaller than the normal adult. The makers of sphygmomanometer cuffs have realised that and today provide a range of cuff sizes that take into account the fact that it is the nature of an infant or child to be physically smaller than an adult.

The example illustrates that when we are trying to establish what is true about children, it is essential to use tools that have been developed with children in mind; tools that reference what is expected in a child. A tool that has been developed for use in adults will usually give some kind of result, and that result might seem plausible. But if what it measures depends on something that is normatively different between adults and children, the results are incorrect as a matter of fact, and any decisions made on the basis of those erroneous estimations can be dangerously wrong.[3] In establishing the value of childness, it is not enough to recognise that the infant is not able to do what an adult can do. That is obviously true, but without prejudging the issue at hand it does not say anything at all about the absolute value of what the infant *can* do. We need to assess the value of the infant's capabilities independently of any reference to what is normal in, or expected from, adults.

4.2   Reasoning Away from Adult-Normativity

The basis of adult-normative reasoning is that the value of the way in which someone enjoys their existence should always be assessed by comparison with the way in which adults do so. Considered as a piece of logic, one 'red flag' is that such thinking quickly leads to a contradiction. Normality is the justification for giving

---

[3] The analogy can, of course, be stretched too far. It turns out, for example, that when blood pressure is accurately measured using appropriately sized cuffs, the normal range in children is genuinely different from that among adults, though not as different as it appears when using the wrong cuff.

full value to the characteristics of adultness, but on adult-normative terms that same yardstick is also the justification for giving no value to the characteristics of childness. Attaching the label 'infant' to an individual human entails certain claims about the things she cannot do, because those are things that no normal human can do as an infant. She is normal because she cannot do them. But if the way *adult* humans sense and interact with the world is the yardstick to determine the way *all* normal humans should sense and interact with the world, the infant is an abnormal human being because she does not sense and interact in a normal human way. But that is not the way in which the infant is, as it were, 'supposed' to sense and interact, so if we regard adultness as the normal state for humans, the infant is both normal and abnormal simultaneously. Infants and children find themselves in a predicament that Tamar Schapiro calls 'normative immaturity'.[4] While the adult is accorded full personal value if he is normal, it is the infant's very normality that assures he is valued less than the adult.

Another 'red flag' is that adult-normativity represents what Beauchamp and Childress call a 'pretheoretical moral position'; in other words, a bias that is already in place before reasoning begins and is therefore in a sense out of the sight of the reasoner herself.[5] Taking such a pretheoretical position reinforces an evaluation that the reasoner has already made, but it does so invisibly. There are various different ways in which normal humans think; if we decide that one of them is more nearly ideal than the others, then the inferiority of the other ways of thinking is already established. It becomes impossible to subject other normal ways of human thinking to any further rational analysis. Worse, once that value judgement has been assimilated into the way society thinks, there is a danger that it comes to be seen as self-evident and becomes self-perpetuating. Charles Darwin's genius was not enough to prevent his lending endorsement to the prevailing societal idea that the way in which women think is inferior to the way in which men think.[6] In defence of his conclusions, Darwin invokes the observation that men achieve more in society: 'The chief distinction in the intellectual powers of the two sexes is shewn by man's attaining to

---

[4] Schapiro, 'What Is a Child?', p. 730. Schapiro goes on to make an argument from Kant that 'Our negative obligation as adults must be to refrain from … treating children as if they belonged to a distinct and permanent underclass. To say that we are not to treat children as if they belonged to a distinct class means that we are not to treat them as anything other than practical agents, creatures who share with us the human problem of finding reasons for action. We are not to treat them as if they were mere objects to be possessed, manipulated, and exploited; nor may we treat them as if they were wild animals, creatures of instinct who have no potential for reason' (Ibid., p. 735).

[5] 'From ancient Hellenic times to the present, we have witnessed pretheoretical moral positions, and motives are at work when groups of people … have been refused a certain social standing on grounds that they lack some property and therefore do not have full moral status'. Beauchamp and Childress, *Principles of Biomedical Ethics*, pp. 81–82.

[6] 'It is generally admitted that with woman the powers of intuition, of rapid perception, and perhaps of imitation, are more strongly marked than in man; but some, at least, of these faculties are characteristic of the lower races, and therefore of a past and lower state of civilization'. Charles Darwin, *The descent of man part III*, eds Adrian J. Desmond and James Moore (London: Penguin Classics, 2017).

a higher eminence, in whatever he takes up, than can woman …'[7] Society at the time was much less likely to grant that sort of 'higher eminence' to women because there was already a prior assumption that the way men think is better, and society rewarded its members for demonstrating that way of thinking. Darwin is judging the quality of all human cognition according to a scale that is primarily attuned to the sorts of thinking that men do well, because those who are encouraged to be interested in the subject (largely men) have judged that way of thinking to be the best way for *all* humans to think. As a result, he fails to realise that the reason women attain less than men in Victorian society is not because there is anything inherently inferior about the way women think, but because the society which determined who attained what eminence was a society which systematically undervalued the things that women can do better than men.[8] Darwin has not realised that he has already presumed the point under contention. Their poor showing intellectually was not indicative of something women couldn't do; it was the result of a value judgement society had already made about the unimportance of what they *could* do. Greater attainment on the part of men reinforced Darwin's belief that men's cognition is better, but in reality it says nothing at all about women's actual ability, because the answer begs the question.

There is the same risk in accepting uncritically the idea that the way in which adults think is the best way for all humans to think. Childness is, of course, less valuable than adultness if one is already committed to the idea that the cognitive capabilities of a normal infant are of less value than those of the normal adult. The basis for that differential evaluation seems to be that the ideal way for all humans to be is to be a normal adult, but that merely expresses in different words the idea that adultness is more valuable than childness, which presupposes the point under contention. In effect, that argument can be stated as: 'Childness is better than adultness, because experiencing life as an adult is better than experiencing it as an infant, which in turn is because adultness is better than childness.'[9] Since we now know

---

[7] Ibid.

[8] For the purposes of the parallel I am drawing here, I am not challenging Darwin's conviction that men and women do think systematically differently, although the claim would be more critically received today than it was among the audience of nineteenth century men whom Darwin was principally addressing. The prevailing view in the twenty-first century is that there probably is a difference (for example, D. M. Greenberg et al., 'Testing the Empathizing-Systemizing theory of sex differences and the Extreme Male Brain theory of autism in half a million people', *Proc Natl Acad Sci U S A,* 115/48 (Nov 27 2018), 12152–57.) but that the variability within such vast numbers of people means that a knowledge of the difference between men *generally* and women *generally* is not at all a valid basis on which to make any judgement about an individual man or woman (Gina Rippon, 'No, that study doesn't prove that men and women think differently', https://www.newstatesman.com/politics/feminism/2018/11/no-study-doesn-t-prove-men-and-women-think-differently, accessed 24th June 2019).

[9] The sense in which Peter Singer uses the term 'infant' in his book *Practical Ethics* illustrates this circular reasoning because it derives from the internal logic of his own argument for infanticide. He uses 'infant' to denote a human who is indifferent to her continuing existence because she is too young to have acquired the cognitive skills that would enable her to prefer to continue to live. Defining the term in that way excludes the possibility that, on Singer's terms, an infant might have

that infants are capable of doing *something* cognitively, adult-normative reasoning represents a pretheoretical judgement that needs to be abandoned if children are to be evaluated properly. As Wall goes on to say: '… if children are to be fully included as members of the human community, some basic sense of "the human" is ultimately required, one that does not silently assume adulthood as its model'.[10]

In order to do so, we first need to uncouple two ideas that we often instinctively conflate; namely, the idea of change over time on the one hand, and progress towards a goal on the other. When we observe the way that something changes over passage of time, we instinctively give that change a narrative that reflects our own values and perceptions. Typically, that narrative is one of progression towards some kind of goal or aspiration. Whether, on observing a housing estate being built on a field, we interpret it as welcome evidence that hitherto useless land is developing into comfortable and affordable accommodation for young families, or distressing evidence that the natural world is degenerating into a mess of concrete, brick and tarmac, depends on whether you are a property developer or an environmentalist. The direction of travel—degeneration on the one hand, development on the other—is determined by one's own values and not simply by what is observed.

The term 'maturation' is in effect inherently an evaluative judgement, because it already implies a sense of having arrived at a point that is in some way better than the point of departure. David Archard suggests that the implication that value augments with age has been the basis in moral philosophy for evaluating a child's status:

> If an adult human's moral status derives from the fact of her being rational, autonomous, and responsible, it follows that a child, which is an unfinished adult, is essentially that which is not yet fully rational, autonomous, or responsible. The 'not yet' is crucial. A child is unlike, say, an animal in lacking capacities and characteristics that it can never acquire. The child is, by contrast, incomplete but open to completion. Indeed, the work of finishing will normally be accomplished by the progress of time. But, although the 'yet' qualifies the 'not' in this crucial manner, it also indicates that what comes later is the fulfilment of a prior lack.[11]

Because infants change into adults over time, it is tempting to assume that the change represents progress towards a goal, and to infer on that basis that it represents an augmentation in value as the individual approaches that goal. The narrative that being a child means being a 'work in progress' may be partly because philosophers are almost always adults. As adults, it is natural for us to assume that the way we are must be the best way for any human to be, and to see the infant and child through that adult-normative lens. One limitation of the acorn metaphor we saw in the last chapter is that it takes for granted that an oak is obviously more valuable

---

full moral value as a person because his definition already entails that she does not. Singer does not commit himself in absolute terms as to when that condition begins or how long it might persist, although he suggests that restricting infanticide to children below a month of age would provide an 'ample safety margin' which implies he expects infancy—on his definition—to persist for more than 4 weeks after birth (Singer, *Practical Ethics*, p. 153).

[10] Wall, *Ethics in light of childhood*, p. 7.

[11] Archard, 'The Oxford Handbook of Practical Ethics', in p. 92.

than an acorn to start with.[12] But that change in value is exactly the point under contention. In order to set aside the potentially prejudicial idea that what is mature is inevitably more nearly ideal than what is immature, a better arboreal metaphor might be the elder tree. On an elder, flowers appear in June, while berries appear in September. It is possible to make wine from both elderflowers and elderberries. Whether the wine-maker considers the elder tree to be fully developed and ready for harvest in June or in September depends on whether his aim is to make elderflower wine or elderberry wine. The value of the bush in June, compared with that in September, depends on which wine he has chosen to make. It does not depend on the fact of three months' having passed, or on the inherent properties of flowers or berries themselves. It is tempting to see flowers as preceding berries, because that sequence aligns best with our sense that things must always progress over time. But if we set that fallacy aside, flowers only precede berries if berries are the desired object. If the purpose of the elder is to make elderflower wine, then berries are prior to flowers. Whether an individual believes that flowers result in berries or vice versa represents a judgement about the purpose of the elder.

The point here is that the idea that childness is valuable primarily because it leads to adultness is deeply embedded in the way we think about childness. But that is because of the narrative adults tell about what is important about human beings. A society that has already decided that full moral status is represented by adultness, and that the defining feature of an infant is that he does not yet possess adultness, must conclude that the moral status of the infant is less than that of the adult. But such a conclusion is no more than the logically inevitable consequence of a particular way of looking at things. It says nothing about the absolute or inherent value of childness.[13] It is no more rational than to suggest that berries are inherently complete or ideal in a way that flowers are not.

There are, of course, some ways in which an adult can reasonably be said to be 'better' than an infant. An adult is, for example, physically stronger and better able to make independent decisions, both of which are useful attributes under certain circumstances. But there are others in which it would be reasonable to suggest it is the *infant* who more closely represents what is ideal. Our observer from outer space

---

[12] For example, Coady states: 'In ordinary discourse, the term "human being" is a kind name like "pig" or "oak tree", and it is simply absurd to think of a pig embryo as a pig, an acorn as an oak tree, or an embryo as a human being' (Coady, 'The common premise for uncommon conclusions'). Coady's point is about rejecting arguments from potential, but his implication is clearly that development from the first word of each pairing to the second represents a change in value, which presumes the point that should be under contention. Coady's reservation presumably concern the term 'being' rather than 'human'.

[13] Moral theologian Ronald Green argues that it would be nonsense to claim that there could be any such objective difference in value between the two states because the break-point between childhood and adulthood has no objective reality: '... biology usually offers not decisive events but only continuous processes of development ... in making status determinations we do not so much identify a point on a developmental continuum where moral respect should be accorded as choose that point'. Ronald M. Green, 'Stem Cell Research: A Target Article Collection Part III – Determining Moral Status', *American journal of bioethics,* 2/1 (2002) p. 20.

might comment that most human beings are born perfectly healthy, but that they deteriorate rapidly, so that after 18 or so years, they have lost much of their capacity for physical healing after injury, and their respiratory and circulatory systems have degenerated to a point where they constantly require high concentrations of oxygen if they are to survive at all. She might follow that up by noting more optimistically that, having reached adulthood, the rate of decline slows down, although it will continue for the next 70 or so years, until death supervenes. Children's sensory and cognitive organs are in first-class condition. If Aristotle is right that a capacity for reason is implied by the existence of the organs necessary for reasoning, there seems to be no a priori reason to assume that the capabilities that characterise childness are any less inherently valuable than those that characterise adultness.

The cognitive changes that take place as childness gives way to adultness, too, should not be taken uncritically to represent maturation towards a developmental goal. It is not a question of progression from a form of awareness that is unfinished, or less than perfect, to one that is perfected. Again, it might even be argued that it represents a form of regression, because spotlight awareness can actually hamper the task of establishing objective truth. One reason that the infant brain is particularly good at soliciting new information is that it has not yet committed itself to prior ideas about the universe as irrevocably as the adult brain has.[14] If human beings were perfectly rational in our attempt to construct explanations for what our sense organs tell us about the world, we would solicit data that disproves our prior hypotheses rather than confirming them. An empirical observation, after all, can be explained by any number of hypotheses, but a hypothesis is unequivocally disproven by a single empirically observed fact that it cannot explain (providing, of course, that fact is what it appears to the observer to be). But humans are not, as a rule, perfectly rational, and outside the disciplines of scientific research almost no one actually does this.[15] We instinctively look for evidence that our explanations are

---

[14] 'Even very young infants have extensive exogenous attention capacities. When they are presented with even highly subtle and conceptually unexpected novel events, they immediately focus their gaze on these events … [A] suggestive picture emerges. When infants and young children process information, there is much less top-down control and inhibition. Infants are sensitive to any information-rich stimuli, not just those stimuli that are relevant to their goals and plans. And because they have much less experience, more stimuli will be information-rich for them than for us. With less top-down inhibition their processing and plasticity will be more distributed and less focused than those of adults'. Gopnik, 'Why babies are more conscious than we are'.

[15] Even within such disciplines it has not always been common practice. The basis of what has come to be called the 'scientific method' was set out in the mid-twentieth century by philosopher of science Sir Karl Popper in his exposition of falsificationism. Popper points out that, when it comes to establishing objective truth, the best that observed evidence can ever achieve is to demonstrate that a hypothesis is wrong. The number of hypotheses that can be constructed to explain what we observe is vast. Since what we observe is only a small part of what actually exists, observation alone cannot tell us which of those many plausible explanations is the true one. But a hypothesis is certainly objectively wrong if it cannot predict or explain what we *do* observe. The distinctiveness of science, according to Popper, is that, unlike mythology, science makes claims that are vulnerable to that sort of disproof: 'Thus my proposal was, and is, that it is this second boldness, together with the readiness to look for tests and refutations, which distinguished "empirical" science from non-science, and especially from pre-scientific myths and metaphysics' (Karl

right, even though the result is often to perpetuate and to crystallise hypotheses objectively that, as a matter of fact, are mis-explanations of reality.

The lantern awareness that characterises childness makes that less likely. It allows infants to see a much greater proportion of the world around them than the more focused way in which normal adults are aware of things most of the time. The sheer amount of new information presenting itself for processing by the infant brain means the infant is less likely to focus on one part of what the infant perceives. The more pedestrian adult brain fails to notice much of what is around it because, on the basis of hypotheses it has constructed beforehand, it has typically already decided what is important and what is not. The result is that babies are less likely than adults to overlook what they perceive. As developmental neuropsychologist Alison Gopnik puts it, 'Babies are more conscious than we [adults] are'.[16] Perhaps adultness should be seen as a form of senescence; a period during which humans begin to lose what is most important, such as depending on others and assessing the world without prejudgement, and find themselves instead having to live largely independently of one another and relying on hypotheses about the universe that in reality are often unreliable.

4.3 Summary

Broadly speaking, the more restricted a moral theory is in its conception of how humans can enjoy being alive, the more likely that theory is to fail to accord personal value where, even on consequentialist terms, such value exists. Adult-normativity represents one such restriction. Taking the position that flourishing as an adult is better than flourishing as an infant or child introduces a systematic bias into medical ethics and represents the same sort of casual depreciation as the Victorians' estimates of women's intellect. Critics of Peter Singer were once unkind

---

R. Popper and Paul Arthur Schilpp, *The philosophy of Karl Popper* (Library of living philosophers; La Salle: Open Court, 1974), pp. 980–81). Popper distances himself from the simplistic logical positivism that characterises some approaches to empiricism. He observes that myths and metaphysics are inherently unprovable, but rejects the conclusion that they are therefore unimportant or untrue. He dismisses, for example, the idea that science disproves theism: 'It may be well to mention at once one important difference between the authors: a difference in religious belief. One of us (Eccles) is a believer in God and the supernatural, while the other (Popper) may be described as an agnostic. Each of us not only deeply respects the position of the other, but sympathizes with it. This difference of opinion should be quite immaterial in our discussion of some of the problems, especially of the purely scientific ones' (Karl R. Popper and John C. Eccles, *The self and its brain* (Berlin/London: Springer International, 1977)).

[16] 'Babies are more conscious than we are. They are ceaselessly and broadly engaged in the kind of information-processing and learning that adults direct only at limited, relevant events. And babies are less subject to the processes that actively cause unconsciousness in adults–inhibition and habituation'. Gopnik, *The Philosophical Baby*. See also Rebecca Nye, *The Child's Curriculum* (Oxford University Press, 2018), p. 139.

enough to suggest that his support for infanticide puts him morally on all fours with the Nazi eugenicists.[17] That is unfair; Singer is saying that infants can be killed, not that they must. But the critics were right that Singer's willingness to end the lives of infants, simply because infants experience their lives in ways that are different from adults, is ultimately no less arbitrary than any other form of preference for one sort of person over another.

During the interval between the extreme childness of infancy, and the extreme adultness of adulthood, a person gradually exchanges some of the capacities of childness for those of adultness. As an infant, a person is good at processing information without prejudice, and at existing effortlessly in dependent relationships; capacities that are important for the kind of biographical narrative the infant needs to construct. Over the course of childhood, a person gains a capacity for thinking analytically in ways that are important for the kind of biographical narrative needed by adults. The capacities of adultness that he acquires increasingly enable him to construct a narrative that is logical and plausible, even if it is not always congruent with what is objectively true. At the same time, however, he gradually loses some of the capacities of childness. His ability to process new information becomes more restricted, so that he tends to interpret data about the world from sense organs on the basis of a prior hypothesis she has already constructed. He begins to make assumptions about himself (for example, that he will continue to exist into the future) and about how others experience the world. If there is no reason to assume the child is progressing towards an ideal simply by getting older, then to privilege adultness over childness is itself no more than an instance of subjective narrative construction. Since the capacities of childness are quite sufficient to allow their possessor to construct narrative, and there are respects in which adulthood represents a form of degeneration, rather than of progression, it is not obvious why adulthood should be seen primarily as the perfection or objective of childhood without taking a pretheoretical moral position that already privileges the capacities of adultness over those of childness. It is intuitively easy for an adult to classify the infant as an incomplete adult, but on the basis of the evidence it would be equally rational to conclude that an adult represents no more than a sort of senescent infant.[18]

In the past, our anthropology of the infant and child orbited a largely adult-normative understanding of ethics. We have allowed our conception of childhood to be shaped by our existing ethical frameworks. What we understood about ethics took as its premise an anthropology of children built around the single ethical idea that, at the end of the day, it is being an adult that really counts. The result, as we have seen, is that bioethicists have been able to defend the idea that infants and children are of lesser value than adults because they cannot live up to that standard.

---

[17] Singer, *Practical Ethics*, p. viii.

[18] Of course, that conclusion is vulnerable to the same arguments in reverse. The point is that there is no logical reason to assume that either set of characteristics (adultness on the one hand, or childness on the other) is inherently more valuable than the other.

But why *should* infants be expected to think like adults, or judged on their inability to do so? Rather than allowing our evaluation of childness to be shaped by what we understand about ethics, we need to ensure that our understanding of ethics is shaped by what we know about the value of childness. That is particularly important in medical ethics, because medical decisions so often necessitate making judgements that rely on an accurate assessment of personal value. Errors in evaluation will certainly result in infants and children experiencing unnecessary suffering. They may even, all too easily, result in the death of an individual who is actively engaged in enjoying her life, simply because she is doing it in a way that the adults around her do not understand or appreciate.

In the light of what we now know about childness, we can begin to ensure that our understanding of ethics in children now begins to orbit a rational and evidence-based anthropology of the infant and child. In the following chapters, I will show that adult-normative evaluations of infants and children have persisted into the moral theories and analytical frameworks that dominate medical ethical discourse in the twenty-first century, and that those adult-normative approaches prevent an unbiased evaluation of the characteristics of childness. Fortunately, I will suggest, technology now provides empirical data about children and their cognitive capacities to which moral philosophers in earlier ages had no access so that, having identified the kind of prejudgement to which adult-normative moral philosophy easily falls prey, we will be in a position to set it aside and to develop instead a rational and coherent account of the value of childness which will enable us properly to evaluate the child *sui generis*.

Bibliography

Archard D. Children. In: LaFollette H, editor. The Oxford handbook of practical ethics. Oxford: Oxford University Press; 2005.

Beauchamp T, Childress J. Principles of biomedical ethics. 6th ed. New York: Oxford University Press; 2009.

Coady CA. The common premise for uncommon conclusions. J Med Ethics. 2013;39(5):284–8.

Darwin C. The descent of man part III (eds. Desmond AJ, Moore J). London: Penguin Classics; 2017.

Gopnik A. Why babies are more conscious than we are. Behav Brain Sci. 2007;30(5–6):503–4.

Gopnik A. The philosophical baby: what children's minds tell us about truth love & the meaning of life. London: Bodley Head; 2009.

Green RM. Stem cell research: a target article collection part III – determining moral status. Am J Bioeth. 2002;2(1):20.

Greenberg DM, et al. Testing the Empathizing-Systemizing theory of sex differences and the Extreme Male Brain theory of autism in half a million people. Proc Natl Acad Sci USA. 2018;115(48):12152–7.

Nye R. The child's curriculum. Oxford University Press; 2018.

Popper KR, Eccles JC. The self and its brain. Berlin/London: Springer International; 1977.

Popper KR, Schilpp PA. The philosophy of Karl Popper, Library of living philosophers. La Salle: Open Court; 1974.

Rippon G. No, that study doesn't prove that men and women think differently. 2019. https://www.newstatesman.com/politics/feminism/2018/11/no-study-doesn-t-prove-men-and-women-think-differently. Accessed 24th June.

Schapiro T. What is a child? Ethics. 1999;109(4):715–38.

Singer P. Practical ethics. New York: Cambridge University Press; 2011.

Wall J. Ethics in light of childhood. Washington, DC: Georgetown University Press; 2010.

Chapter 5
Childness in Principlism

Generally speaking, doctors are healthy, wealthy and well-educated, while patients are unwell and often vulnerable. In order to redress the inevitable power imbalance and to avoid exploitation, society expects doctors to behave according to a carefully considered moral code. There have been many such codes down the centuries. Perhaps the most famous is the Hippocratic Oath, which was articulated in the fifth century BCE and, through a series of vows that a doctor makes to the gods, explains that a 'good doctor' should be humble, honest, skilled and compassionate. Most doctors no longer swear the Oath, although even today its influence is often clear in how societies mandate that medicine should be practised.[1]

While it is a useful touchstone for professionalism, however, the Oath does not function as a day-to-day guide to inform clinicians' decisions in the specific ethical quandaries they encounter while caring for patients. The ethical question that usually faces a clinician is not whether or not she should be the sort of person who wants the best for her patient; that is taken as read. When a clinician asks an ethical question, the advice she is usually looking for is what specific action she should take in order to achieve that best. The authors of Principlism aim to offer clinicians just such a useful practical guide. Principlism was first set out in 1977 by Thomas Beauchamp and James Childress, and 50 years later it remains the dominant paradigm for medical ethics among clinicians, at least in the West.[2] In most medical schools, the 'four principles' approach of Principlism is the basis for systematic training in medical ethics, and most clinicians will be as familiar with the terms

---

[1] B. Green, 'Use of the Hippocratic or other professional oaths in UK medical schools in 2017: practice, perception of benefit and principlism', *BMC Res Notes,* 10/1 (Dec 29 2017), 777. See, for example, General Medical Council, *Good Medical Practice* (London: General Medical Council, 2023).

[2] Quoted in T. L. Beauchamp, 'Principlism and its alleged competitors', *Kennedy Inst Ethics J,* 5/3 (Sep 1995), 181–98.

R. Hain, *Childness and the Myth of the Unfinished Human,*
https://doi.org/10.1007/978-3-032-12111-0_5

'beneficence', 'non-maleficence', 'interests', 'autonomy' and 'justice' as they are with concepts of 'drug bioavailability', 'distribution' and 'elimination half-life'.

The term 'Principlism' itself, though convenient, is perhaps regrettable because it can be taken to imply that Beauchamp and Childress are aiming to set out a single coherent moral theory. That is not true. The aim of the authors of Principlism is pragmatic. Moral theories can be complex, recondite, elliptical and abstract, and it would be difficult for a busy clinician to appeal to any one specific theory in order to resolve the moral quandaries that arise in everyday practice. Principlism is designed to provide a structure for clinicians' ethical thinking about the practical quandaries that busy clinicians frequently face. Its objective is to provide practical advice that is readily accessible to clinicians and can be assimilated 'in the heat of battle', but is at the same time ethically sound and explainable by careful moral reasoning. Rather than a moral theory in itself, Principlism is a heuristic that brings together a 'framework of norms' derived from several different moral philosophical theories.[3] It accordingly represents: '… clusters of principles [which] derive from considered judgements in the common morality and professional traditions in health care, particularly medicine and nursing' and its authors' aim is to '… develop, specify, and balance these principles'.[4] Principlism is the visible outline of the landscape of contemporary medical ethics, but it is shaped by a substratum formed of many different moral ideas. Its sources are eclectic, and Beauchamp and Childress draw critically and selectively on several sorts of theory, particularly deontology, consequentialism and virtue ethics.

5.1 Principlism and Childness

The framework that Beauchamp and Childress present summarises the moral theories that underpin medical ethics by means of four sorts of obligation that its authors describe as principles. Beneficence and non-maleficence respectively describe the physician's duty to do good and her duty to avoid harm. While there are important differences between them, both duties express an obligation to act in a way that promotes the well-being of the individual and, in practice, they are often considered together as a duty to act in a way that will further a patient's interests. The duty to respect others' autonomy expresses an obligation to facilitate a patient's own agency, primarily by refusing to intervene in the face of competent refusal but also by actively soliciting, and giving appropriate weight to, a patient's preferences in medical decisions that affect her.[5] The principle of justice is usually taken to refer to

---

[3] Beauchamp and Childress, *Principles of Biomedical Ethics*, pp. 17, 25.

[4] Thomas Beauchamp and James Childress, *Principles of Biomedical Ethics* (6th edn.; New York: Oxford University Press, 2009), p. 25.

[5] Beauchamp, 'Principlism and its alleged competitors', p. 103.

an obligation to be fair; that is, ensuring that all patients are given equal value and that healthcare resources are utilised equitably.

Principlism asserts the inherent value of a child on grounds that are largely deontological. Its authors suggest that everyone in society agrees that certain obligations are explained by relationships. The relationship between the moral patient and the moral agent expresses an agent's duty to care for others, and as such it also represents an explanation as to why such obligations exist at all. The root of a doctor's obligation to concern herself with a patient's interests is the relationship between moral agent (the person deciding what action to take) and moral patient (the person to whom the action is done).[6] Some relationships inherently obligate the agent to act in a way that will further the interests of the moral patient. Beauchamp and Childress characterise those as: '… very close moral relationships' that are illustrated by '… contracts or the ties of family or friendship'.[7] Other relationships carry no such obligation. The agent's duty to concern herself with another's interests depends on what the subject of moral action should expect from the moral agent, which, for the purposes of ethical reasoning, is what defines their relationship.[8] Principlism considers that the relationship between parents and children is an obvious illustration. Parents' care of an infant or child provides such a clear example of the 'contracts or ties of family or friendship', which define such obligations that, in their view, it does not need further explanation:

> Specific beneficence is directed at specific parties, such as children, friends, and patients, whereas general beneficence is directed beyond these special relationships to all persons … *virtually everyone agrees* that all persons are obligated to act, in certain circumstances, in the interests of their children …[9]

In other words, everyone already agrees that it is inherent in the nature of the relationship between parent and child that the former should care for the latter, and that the existence of that relationship is enough to account for the obligation on a parent to further the interests of the child. That is equally true in respect of a child at any stage, including infancy, because the obligation is not connected to the characteristics of the child herself. Relationship, in the sense that is held by Principlism to be morally relevant, is defined by the moral duty that the relationship expresses. The fact of shared genetic material is epiphenomenal and, although such duties typically occur in the context of people who are biologically connected through common DNA, for moral purposes it is not that connection that defines relationship. The obligations of a woman to her adopted daughter are precisely the same, for example, as her obligations to her

---

[6] Specific beneficence is directed at specific parties, such as children, friends, and patients, whereas general beneficence is directed beyond these special relationships to all persons. Beauchamp and Childress, *Principles of Biomedical Ethics*, pp. 199–200.

[7] Ibid., p. 202.

[8] Beauchamp and Childress use the Biblical parable of the Good Samaritan to illustrate the point. The Samaritan was not known to the traveller and there was nothing in their relationship that required him to care for the traveller. His attention to the traveller's interests was therefore supererogatory, rooted in compassion rather than in obligation or duty (Ibid., p. 198).

[9] Beauchamp and Childress, *Principles of Biomedical Ethics*, pp. 199–200. (Authors' italics).

biological daughter. The terms 'mother' and 'daughter' denote that such obligations exist, and for moral purposes that is the full extent of their meaning.[10]

By invoking the moral power of obligations entailed in relationships, an argument from relationships offers infants and children some protection from the risk of being undervalued on the basis of their cognitive shortcomings. On those terms, the obligatory nature of the specific principle of beneficence does not depend on any normative criterion of personhood in the beneficiary of moral action. The infant or child's inability to reason logically, for example, does not have to mean that the infant or child lacks personal value, because the agent's obligation to be concerned with the child's interests does not directly depend on such an ability. By insisting on deontological grounds that adults should care for children, an argument from relationships goes some way to attenuating the practical risks attendant on privileging adultness over childness. Principlism's deontological account of personal value in infants and children represents an important 'work-around' to adult-normative thinking in medical ethics.

But it is not a fix. Ethicist and paediatrician Paul Baines points out that none of the four principles applies straightforwardly to paediatrics.[11] His concern is that the principles have been formulated with adults in mind and do not easily translate to the case of children. Although Baines does not use the term 'adult-normative', he recognises that the assumptions on which the principles are based reference values that are characteristic of adults rather than children, and that without an acknowledgement of that bias there is some danger in the way the principles might be applied to ethical quandaries concerning children. He notes, for example, that an obligation to respect autonomy is often thought to be more important than the other four principles but that its relevance to most children is restricted and that it is of no relevance at all to infants. There is a risk that Principlism gives such weight to an obligation to respect autonomy that the clinician will feel under pressure to cast around for someone whose autonomy he can respect, which in practice usually means the child's parents. From there it is a short step to concluding that a medical decision over a child is right merely because it is what her parents prefer.

----

[10]The relationship of the paediatrician to the infant can also be described as a contract, so that an argument from relationships explains why a doctor, as well as a child's parents, should attend to the interests of an infant or child. The existence of that therapeutic relationship is, in effect, a contract which explains an obligation for a paediatrician to further the interests of a patient who is an infant or child. Elsewhere, Childress endorses Paul Ramsey's assertion that the relationship between doctor and patient is best described as a 'covenant of loyalty'. James F. Childress, 'Protestant Perspectives on Informed Consent (Particularly in Research Involving Human Participants)', *Fordham Urban Law Journal,* 30/1 art 11 (2002), 187–205. See also Paul Ramsey, 'The enforcement of morals: nontherapeutic research on children', *The Hastings Center report,* 6/4 (Aug 1976), 21–30. Ramsey characterises a doctor's relationship with children as one of trust: '… faithfulness-claims which a child, simply by being a normal or a sick or a dying child, places upon us and medical care' and concludes uncompromisingly that: 'We should expect no significant exceptions to this canon of faithfulness to the child'. Paul Ramsey, *The Patient as Person: Explorations in Medical Ethics* (Yale University Press, 2002).

[11]P. Baines, 'Medical ethics for children: applying the four principles to paediatrics', *Journal of Medical Ethics,* 34/3 (March 1, 2008), 141–45.

Beauchamp and Childress have not dispensed with the idea that adultness is more valuable than childness. They have not proposed an anthropology of the child that is not adult-normative. Rather than developing a foundational account of the value of the childness on which to construct an explanation for the value of an infant and child, Beauchamp and Childress have relied on societal norms about how adults 'should' treat infants and children. They have observed that everyone agrees that the nature of their relationship means that parents owe a special duty of care to their own infants, but have not provided a reasoned explanation as to why, or even whether, that is something everyone *should* agree.

What's more, the fact that 'virtually everyone' agrees does not guarantee that they will always do so. While Principlism is right to suggest that, at this point in history, most societies largely concede that an agent has specific obligations to the infant, even today that agreement is not universal. Many utilitarian consequential-ists, in particular, would dissent because there is a tension between the ethical sig-nificance of family ties and the importance of the utilitarian principle of impartiality. See Bentham's impartial observer and Sidgwick's dispassionate and impersonal universe impose on the agent a general obligation to prevent harm, providing moral risk, cost or burden to the agent is not significant. But they do not offer a reason for considering that that obligation should be greater in respect of some parties -even one's own children- than others. Chinese sage Mo Tzu argued in around 400 BC that, in an ideal world, the compassion of parents for their own children would be no different from their concern for the children of others.[12] Contemporary utilitarian philosopher James Rachels considers several possible moral objections to Mo's proposition but rejects all of them and concludes that there is little theoretical justi-fication for bias towards one's own children. At the same time, he reluctantly acknowledges that the belief that there should be such a bias—what he calls 'the most common view'—is so strong and so widely held that, in practice, a preference for the interests of one's own children is inevitable.[13]

Singer, too, rejects the moral power of relationships. Beauchamp and Childress illustrate the difference between obligatory and ideal beneficence using the parable of the good Samaritan.[14] Singer sees their parable and raises them his own story of the shallow pond, first published some years before *Practical Ethics*: '… if I am walking past a shallow pond and see a child drowning in it, I ought to wade in and pull the child out. This will mean getting my clothes muddy, but this is insignificant, while the death of the child would presumably be a very bad thing'.[15] The moral responsibility of an agent to save the life of the child in front of her, he suggests, is no greater than her

---

[12] James Rachels, *Can ethics provide answers? and other essays in moral philosophy* (Lanham; London: Rowman & Littlefield, 1997).

[13] Rachels suggests that a reasonable compromise is to adopt a position of 'partial bias', in which parents prioritise the interests of their own children over those of others, but nevertheless regard the interests of other children as material and important (Ibid., pp. 231–32).

[14] Luke 10:25–37 (quoted in Beauchamp and Childress, *Principles of Biomedical Ethics*, p. 198).

[15] Peter Singer, 'Famine, affluence and morality', *Philosophy and Public Affairs,* 1/1 (1972), 229–43. Singer's interpolation of the word 'presumably' is noteworthy.

responsibility to save the life of a child who is dying of starvation on another continent whom he has ever met.[16] Singer appears to be stating something self-evident here, namely that morality is not related to the distance between agent and moral patient. Proximity itself is a patently arbitrary basis on which to prioritise the interests of some parties over others. An agent might well feel a special duty to intervene to further the interests of a child whom he can see drowning in front of him, but that is not simply because the child is close by. It is on the basis that, because of her proximity, he knows that the child needs help, and he is in a position to offer it. Singer argues that those practical considerations are all that make a relationship relevant.[17] He does not distinguish physical proximity from social proximity (a convenient synonym for relationship), because, according to a consequentialist account, that distinction is unnecessary. The agent's physical closeness to the child, and her knowledge of what needs to be done to further the child's interests, are what define their relationship. To say the agent has a relationship with a particular party means no more than that the party is physically proximate, and that her needs are clearly known to the agent. There is nothing in the argument that Singer is making about 'a neighbour's child ten yards away' that is not equally true about the agent's own child. The shallow-pond story—at least, as Singer expounds it in its original form—illustrates a utilitarian view that society is wrong if it thinks that parents are entitled to be biased in favour of their own children simply because of the relationship between them.

Despite such consequentialist protests, for the time being, Beauchamp and Childress do seem to be justified in their belief that 'virtually everyone agrees' that an adult's obligation to a child is determined primarily by their relationship. Even Singer finds it difficult to remain consistent with the idea that relationships are of no moral relevance. When he re-tells the shallow-pond parable in *Practical Ethics*, he makes an important modification to the original which had appeared some years earlier:

---

[16] 'It makes no moral difference whether the person I can help is a neighbor's child ten yards from me or a Bengali whose name I shall never know, ten thousand miles away … I do not think I need to say much in defense of the refusal to take proximity and distance into account. The fact that a person is physically near to us, so that we have personal contact with him, may make it more likely that we *shall* assist him, but this does not show that we *ought* to help him rather than another who happens to be further away' (Ibid., p. 2).

[17] 'Admittedly, it is possible that we are in a better position to judge what needs to be done to help a person near to us than one far away, and perhaps also to provide the assistance we judge to be necessary. If this were the case, it would be a reason for helping those near to us first' (Ibid). Singer also argues that in these days of rapid information exchange, it is no longer reasonable to link knowledge of a party's need with physical proximity to the party. His rejection on utilitarian grounds of the moral relevance of proximity in this respect depends on his belief that technology now makes the needs of all children equally knowable by the agent. Even if that rather unlikely premise were granted, the fact that the needs are potentially knowable is not the point, even on utilitarian grounds. What is relevant is whether or not they are *actually* known to the agent. Irrespective of the state of technology, it is much more likely that the agent will know the needs of a child who is physically proximate, or with whom an agent has a biological relationship. It may be for that reason that, although Singer recapitulates the earlier 'shallow pond' parable in *Practical Ethics* (pp. 385–387), his emphasis is no longer on dismissing the moral relevance of proximity but on the principle of comparable moral importance.

> On my way to give a lecture, I pass a shallow ornamental pond and notice that a small child
> has fallen in and is in danger of drowning. *I look around to see where the parents, or
> babysitter, are, but to my surprise, I see that there is no one else around. It seems that it is
> up to me to make sure that the child doesn't drown.*[18]

Before concluding that it is his duty to rescue the child, this latter Singer has first
established that there is no one around—no parent or babysitter—whose relationship with the child is such that it is *they* who should do the rescuing. There seems no
obvious utilitarian reason why the character Singer should do this, since he himself
is already aware of the child's need and is in a position to address it. Like 'virtually
everyone' else, he seems here to take Rachels' most common view that the relationship between parent or carer and child confers on them an obligatory duty of beneficence that exceeds that of a stranger.

Nevertheless, the global agreement about relationships on which Principlism relies
for its protection of infants and children should not be taken for granted. While
Beauchamp and Childress and Rachels are undoubtedly correct that at this point in history society shows no sign of expecting parents not to be biased in favour of their own
children, that agreement is ultimately rooted only in social convention and, like all
social conventions, could change unless there is a persuasive account of the value of
infants and children that derives from a moral anthropology of the child in which the
value of a child does not rely wholly on society's current belief that caring for infants
and children is simply what parents should do. Even if 'virtually everyone' agrees that
parents should be biased in favour of their own children, that consensus is a slender
reed on which infants and children should not have to rely for their value to be protected.

5.1.1   Interests: Beneficence and Non-Maleficence

There is a distinction between the obligation to avoid harming someone by acting
against her best interests (non-maleficence) and an obligation to help them by acting
in her best interests (beneficence). Non-maleficence states the bare minimum obligation on doctors; that they should at least make their patients no worse.[19]
Beneficence, on the other hand, describes a duty to act in a way that actively makes
patients better. On the face of it, the obligations of beneficence and non-maleficence
are self-evident and seem to need no further explanation. According to Principlism,

---

[18] Singer, *Practical Ethics*, p. 385. My italics.

[19] Hippocrates too enjoined physicians, if they could not help cure a disease, then '… at least, [to]
do no harm'. Hippocrates, *Epidemics* 1:11 (quoted in Beauchamp and Childress, *Principles of
Biomedical Ethics*, p. 207). The principle of non-maleficence imposes negative obligations that are
impartial, in that the agent can fulfil them in respect of everyone in the world simultaneously simply by not doing anything at all, and can therefore provide moral reasons for prohibiting certain
actions, if necessary through legislation. The extent to which a moral agent should act in order to
prevent harm is logically limited only by the extent of the impact of other (positive) outcomes of
that action and therefore depends on an assessment of net interests.

actions that are beneficent beneficence can encompass not only conduct that is morally obligatory, but also conduct that would be ideal, but should not be enforced. Unfortunately, in practice almost every therapeutic intervention in medicine carries the certainty that the patient will experience both harm and benefit.[20] At the time a medication is prescribed, or a procedure is carried out, any physician knows that her action will have multiple outcomes that are certain. She also knows that several further outcomes are possible, the probability of each of which can be estimated even though they cannot be known with certainty. It would be highly unusual for all the certain or possible consequences of an intervention to work equally for a patient's good. It is always even possible (through something that is unknown to the doctor or simply through the operation of chance) that the action will, after all, cause significant harm that outweighs any benefit. In proceeding with the intervention, a doctor is making a judgement that, on balance, the harms are likely to be outweighed by the benefits. The basis for her judgement is what the doctor knows and understands about that intervention. But even as she makes that judgement, the physician also knows that there is a chance that the intervention will do this particular patient a significant harm that outweighs the good.

In an attempt to accommodate that complexity, in clinical practice the concept of interests is usually taken to refer to the net benefit and harm that is expected by the agent to result from a decision. So, for example, when a hospital Clinical Ethics Committee asserts that intubation and ventilation of a seriously ill child are 'not in the child's interests', they do not mean to suggest that the intervention offers no benefits. Rather, they mean it will cause inevitable harms of discomfort and fear, which will threaten the child's well-being to a degree that they believe is likely to exceed its benefits. A decision is said to be 'in a patient's interests' if, on balance, it will do more good than harm.[21]

Because they are not constrained by a single moral theory, it is open to Beauchamp and Childress to consider the nature of value in a variety of different ways. They acknowledge that a consequentialist calculation of net interests is relevant to the obligations of a duty of beneficence, but also appeal to the

---

[20]That is not just because a single therapeutic intervention can encompass several individual actions. Even a single action will usually carry the possibility of many different consequences, some of which are harmful. Patients—and sometimes even ethicists—wrongly assume that benefits and harms are alternatives to one another ('There is a 90% chance this drug will offer benefit, so there must be a 10% chance it will do harm'). Pharmacological effects are not a 'zero sum game' because harms and benefits are separate; they not mutually exclusive by pharmacology, and the reality is that the probability of benefit is largely unconnected to the probability of harm except to the extent that there is a lengthy and robust process that prevents drugs being sold unless the probability of benefit relative to harm is very high.

[21]In legal parlance, 'best interests' refers to the single course of action in relation to a patient that a Court has instructed. In clinical practice, however, the terms 'interests' and 'best interests' are often used interchangeably. That use is misleading, because it implies that the only morally permissible course of action is the one that ensures the greatest excess of benefit over harm. In reality, there are often several courses of action which plausibly offer enough excess of benefit over harm to make them permissible.

deontological demands of relationship. Both are important; even if the nature of their relationship is enough to account for the fact that a doctor has a duty to a patient, it does not set out the specific obligations that result from that duty and so is not action-guiding on its own. In order for the doctor to know how she should act in response to her obligation to further the interests of her patient, it is necessary for her to understand what the impact of her intervention is likely to be.[22] The obligation on a doctor to concern herself with a patient's interests is on grounds that are consequential as well as deontological.

5.1.2   *Interests and Childness*

It might seem that the concept of interests applies in infants and children in a perfectly straightforward way. 'Interests', on the terms used in this book, refers to the excess of benefit over harm that accrues to an individual as a result of moral action. Since no one disputes that the infant or child can experience benefit and harm, 'interests' seems to represent something that needs no particular or complex specification to medical ethics in infants and children.

Perhaps the greatest difficulty that an adult-normative approach to interests presents to infants and children is that it can restrict the way in which bioethics considers interests in the first place. Our idea of interests has been shaped by adult-normative thinking and, while the fundamental idea of interests itself presents no difficulties to an age-neutral account of medical ethics in children, the way in which interests are usually understood in ethical discourse can restrict our understanding of what interests might 'look like' in infants and children. Some of the ways in which adults and children differ from one another make it likely that what we understand to be interests will look quite different. Viewed through an adult-normative lens, for example, an individual's interests are usually served by an action that facilitates the exercise of rational autonomy based on a rational understanding of the outcome. That is because logical reason, independence and 'futurity' (an understanding that one will continue to exist into the future) are all capacities that characterise adultness. Those same actions would not serve the interests of an infant or young child, because childness is characterised by a way of appreciating the universe that is often non-rational, is built around the child's dependence on others, and as far as we know represents the child's present

---

[22] Peter Singer asserts that the extent to which a moral agent should act in order to prevent harm is logically limited only by the extent of the impact of other (positive) outcomes of that action: 'A plausible principle that would support the judgement that I ought to pull the child out is this: if it is in our power to prevent something very bad happening, without thereby sacrificing anything of comparable moral significance, we ought to do it. This principle seems uncontroversial. It will obviously win the assent of consequentialists; but non-consequentialists should accept it too, because the injunction to prevent what is bad applies only when nothing comparably significant is at stake'. Singer, *Practical Ethics*, p. 386.

experience and sensations rather than relying on speculation about what might happen in the future. There are, in short, obvious ways in which an action that promotes the flourishing of a normal adult would fail to do so in a normal infant or child and might even actively undermine the latter's flourishing. While the concept of interests itself needs no specification in the light of childness—interests are just as relevant to moral deliberation concerning an infant as they are to moral deliberation concerning an adult—the ways in which the moral agent should conceive of those interests are different in a human who exhibits childness, and therefore so are the practical ways in which a moral agent should value her by attending to those interests.

A second difficulty is that, on adult-normative terms, interests are always annexed to an individual. When a decision needs to be made on the basis of a balance of benefits and harms, the benefits and harms in question are those of the individual patient. That is not to say the interests of others are unimportant to the agent's decision, but those interests too are annexed to specific other individuals. While it might sometimes be challenging in practice to disentangle them, an individual's interests are always at least hypothetically separable from the interests of other people. That separability is connected to the individual's capacity for rational autonomy.[23]

Childness, however, is characterised by connection with others, not by independence or isolation from them. A characteristic of childness is that the locus of child's sense of self is not restricted to herself, but in the network of relationships in which the infant knows herself to exist. That intersubjective nature of childness means that the interests of an infant or child are not always separable from the interests of those around her, especially her parents. Some of the infant's interests may have no reality that is separable from the interests of others. There are some interests that do not belong wholly to the infant, for example, or wholly to her parent, but to the dyad of infant and parent together.

The inherently intersubjective nature of interests in childness is of practical importance when it comes to medical ethics in children. There may be an academic sense in which it is the child who is the sole patient of the paediatrician, so that the interests of the child's parents are not material to any judgement the paediatrician may make. Most would, however, consider that doctors have a duty to care for people, and since the paediatrician is a doctor she must also have a secondary concern for the interests of the child's parents. That imposes an obligation to balance the benefits and harms of a proposed action in a way that is in the net interests of all the parties, but acknowledges a greater obligation to the child than to her parents. Such balancing requires the doctor to separate the interests of the child from those of the parents in order to weigh them up against one another. But a doctor cannot simply resolve the relevant interests into those of individuals in order to prioritise the interests of the child over parents, because the interests of the dyad

---

[23] Beauchamp and Childress, *Principles of Biomedical Ethics*, p. 171.

(infant + infant's parent) are not the same as (the interests of the infant) + (the interests of the infant's parent).

Finally, some of the relevant interests of infants and very young children cannot be known. Relatively few of the important differences between the nature of adults and the nature of children relate to what we can call 'objective' interests. Other than size, the physical differences between children and adults are largely trivial and are easily accommodated when it comes to evaluating moral action in medicine. The judgement as to whether or not antibiotics are in a patient's interest, for example, depends on the presence or absence of evidence for infection. It does not depend on knowing whether the patient is an adult or a child. The obligations of beneficence, however, are not restricted to objective medical interests of that sort. While the chance of recovery from sepsis can be inferred without knowing the perspective or preferences of the individual patient, the terms 'harm' and 'benefit' (or 'interests') go beyond that sort of observable phenomenon to include benefits or harms that result from the individual's own perspective on the world, and the personal preferences that result from that perception. To know those 'subjective' interests, the agent must know the person who holds them. When he goes shopping, a husband does not need to know anything about his wife's likes and dislikes to know that he needs to provide her with food, because not starving is an objective interest that is inseparable from her existing at all. But he buys *particular* foods because he knows she likes them. Eating those foods rather than others is an expression of her subjective preferences. Those preferences are relevant to her well-being, and in order to promote it her husband must know something about them. Subjective interests are germane in Principlism, both because they contribute to a utilitarian calculus and because they explain certain specific obligations that fall out of duties. Emotional, psychological and existential dimensions represent interests in Principlism which may be just as important to the patient as objective or commensurable contributors to well-being.

But childness makes them very difficult to know.[24] A restricted ability to communicate subjective experiences to others is a defining characteristic of childness even though it is not limited to infants and children. It is a practical difficulty, perhaps, rather than a moral one. But it is a practical difficulty that appears insurmountable with current technology. It means that, in infants and young children, interests can be relevant—even central—to making an ethically correct decision, without

---

[24] Even in adults, it can be difficult for an agent to infer anything meaningful about the subjective well-being of someone else. An individual's sense of well-being will often correlate only poorly with objective outcomes that are observable and seem intuitively relevant, such as personal wealth, physical health or even political freedom. Patients highly value physical health, for example, and many of the healthcare decisions they take when they are healthy are predicated on the assumption that their well-being in the future will depend critically on how well they are able to function physically. When their physical health is actually eroded, however, patients typically report remarkably little reduction in their well-being. M. A. Echteld et al., 'Changes in and correlates of individual quality of life in advanced cancer patients admitted to an academic unit for palliative care', *Palliat Med,* 21/3 (Apr 2007), 199–205, M. A. Echteld et al., 'Quality of life change and response shift in patients admitted to palliative care units: a pilot study', *Palliat Med,* 19/5 (Jul 2005), 381–8.

being definitely knowable to the moral agent. While we wait for advances that will enable us to access the experiences of those who cannot talk, the agent who wishes to treat the infant correctly is faced with the fact that she has interests that are relevant to how adults should treat her, and yet cannot be directly known.

5.1.3   *Respect for Autonomy*

Modern conceptions of personal autonomy in medical ethics flow both from Kant's notion of freedom to act rationally, and from John Mill's notion of freedom from interference by others.[25] The word 'autonomy' originally described city-states that were considered so well-governed locally that they did not need to submit themselves to the law of the state. It was not used to denote a characteristic of persons until the eighteenth century, when Jean-Jacques Rousseau suggested that what was true of city-states was also true of persons; that is, they did not need to be governed by someone else (always providing they were capable of governing themselves well) and so it would be morally wrong to impose such external government on them.[26]

Although the word 'autonomy' does not appear in Kant, it readily attaches to one of his central ideas, namely that what distinguishes a person from a thing is a capacity for agency. A person can choose to do something; she can make plans and can decide to act in accordance with reason, while an object can only have something done to it. An object can be used as a means to achieve a person's ends, but another person should not.[27] Modern understanding of autonomy often emphasises voluntariness; that is, the extent to which a person is both able to decide to act and to carry out that act without the influence of other people. A Kantian idea of autonomy, on the other hand, also expresses certain restrictions. For Kant, behaving correctly is a matter of reason, and a Kantian concept of autonomy consists not only in having the freedom to act in accordance with the moral law, but also in

---

[25] Mill rarely used the term 'autonomy'. Philosopher Onora O'Neill suggests that, for Mill, the term was irredeemably tainted by its association with Kant's cognitive insistence on a link with reason Onora O'Neill, *Autonomy and trust in bioethics* (Gifford lectures; Cambridge: Cambridge University Press, 2002), p. 30.

[26] 'For to be driven by appetite alone is slavery, and obedience to the law one has prescribed to oneself is liberty'. Jean-Jacques Rousseau, *Social Contract*, Book I, chapter VIII, Sect 3.

[27] 'Thus the worth of all objects to be acquired through our action is always conditioned. The beings whose existence rests not on our will but on nature nevertheless have, if they are beings without reason, only a relative worth as means, and are called things; rational beings, by contrast, are called persons, because their nature already marks them out as ends in themselves, i.e., as something that may not be used merely as means, hence to that extent limits all arbitrary choice (and is an object of respect)'. Kant, Wood, and Schneewind, *Groundwork for the Metaphysics of Morals*, p. 46.

choosing rationally to submit oneself to it.[28] In practice, such rational deliberation does not always obviously guide human decisions. People often passionately want something that will, beyond any reasonable doubt, do them more harm than good. Linking autonomy so firmly with reason leaves open a question of whether an action is permissible if it is unwise or irrational. John Mill responds in the name of freedom that it should be allowed because it should not be stopped. The key issue, according to Mill, is not what reason requires a moral agent to do, but what it prevents her from doing. Over-riding the freely-made decisions of others, he argued, can only be justified to the extent that reason indicates it is unavoidable in order to help them.[29]

Beauchamp and Childress suggest that among the many and varied understandings of autonomy there is a thread of meaning that is generally agreed in medical ethics. Personal autonomy is, they suggest: '… at minimum, self-rule that is free from both controlling interference by others and from limitations, such as inadequate understanding, that prevent meaningful choice. The autonomous individual acts freely in accordance with a self-chosen plan'.[30] The cognitive capacities that explain why an individual is not an object are those that are necessary for reasoning, such as memory, logic and verbal ability. Possession of those cognitive capacities has acquired considerable evaluative power over the years, and, in the twenty-first century, there are procedural criteria for demonstrating that a human individual possesses them. Beauchamp and Childress consider that the normal human possesses those capacities, so that the doctor's obligation to respect autonomy is simply correlative to a right on the part of patients for those capacities to be respected where they are present.[31]

---

[28] 'Every thing in nature works in accordance with laws. Only a rational being has the faculty to act in accordance with the representation of laws, i.e., in accordance with principles, or a will. Since for the derivation of actions from laws reason is required, the will is nothing other than practical reason' (Ibid., p. 29).

[29] 'If either a public officer or any one else saw a person attempting to cross a bridge which had been ascertained to be unsafe, and there were no time to warn him of his danger, they might seize him and turn him back without any real infringement of his liberty; for liberty consists in doing what one desires, and he does not desire to fall into the river'. (John Stuart Mill, 'Chapter V. Applications', in W.L. Courtney (ed.), *On Liberty* (London and Felling-on-Tyne, New York and Melbourne: The Walter Scott Publishing Co., Ltd., 1901)). Mill and his followers had a low threshold for concluding that an action is coercive. Isaiah Berlin points out that they considered the restricting influence of prevailing opinion and even of democratic government to be forms of tyranny (Isaiah Berlin, *Two concepts of liberty: an inaugural lecture delivered before the University of Oxford on 31 October 1958* (Oxford: Clarendon Press, 1958), p. 27).

[30] Beauchamp and Childress, *Principles of Biomedical Ethics*, pp. 99–100.

[31] Ibid., p. 107.

5.1.4   Autonomy and Childness

Principlism understands autonomy in medical practice as self-rule on the part of a patient. 'Respect for autonomy' refers to the correlative moral obligation for a doctor to give appropriate weight to the preferences that a patient expresses over her own treatment. That qualifier 'appropriate' is important; the weight that should given to demands for interventions that are unnecessary is light. The correct response to a patient with a viral illness who demands antibiotics that are unnecessary and potentially dangerous, for example, is to set it aside. The doctor is under no obligation to offer harm to a patient simply because the patient has requested it. The weight of a patient's preference *not* to have an intervention, on the other hand, is so great that the authority of her refusal prevails even over her own interests—*providing the individual possesses the cognitive capacities to understand the consequences of that refusal.* Those cognitive capacities do not characterise childness; indeed, a defining characteristic of childness is a lack of the sort of faculty for calculative logic that self-rule demands. Childness alone confers on the individual a status as an undeveloped agent that has even been described as 'deviant'.[32]

Neither Kant's understanding of moral agency nor Mill's understanding of liberty easily accommodates children. Beauchamp and Childress exclude infants from treatment under this principle, using the word 'childish' specifically to describe an individual who can legitimately be coerced.[33] Beauchamp and Childress object to a theory of moral status and duty based on cognitive criteria.[34] But the basis for that objection is not entirely clear. Childness positively facilitates dependence; far from being free from the influence of others, the normal mode of decision-making for a child is to delegate the task to adults.

Principlism and utilitarianism share the same adult-normative assumption that there is only one meaningful form of autonomy, and that it is the kind of rational independence demonstrated—in the breach, if not always in the observance—by normal adults: 'The autonomous individual acts freely in accordance with a self-chosen plan, analogous to the way an independent government manages its territories and sets its policies'.[35] The capacities of childness do not permit autonomy, so Principlism excludes infants from the physicians' obligation to respect autonomy on the same grounds as utilitarian consequentialists do; namely, that without radically re-conceiving what we mean by autonomy, there is no way in which the infant

---

[32] 'Kantian ideal theory does indeed presuppose that the social world is made up exclusively of developed agents. But in doing so, the theory provides a standard relative to which certain agents can count as undeveloped. It is by defining this deviant status more precisely and by working out its implications that we come to see what an ethic of adult-child relations would entail'. Tamar Schapiro, 'What Is a Child?', *Ethics,* 109/4 (1999), 715–38 p. 732.

[33] Beauchamp and Childress, *Principles of Biomedical Ethics*, p. 134.

[34] Ibid., pp. 72–73.

[35] Ibid., pp. 99–100.

can meaningfully possess it.[36] Their explanation for nevertheless endorsing the argument from marginal cases is essentially pragmatic; it is that any other conclusion would result in a moral theory that fails to protect the vulnerable:

> … every major cognitive criterion of moral status (intelligence, agency, self-consciousness, etc.) excludes some nonautonomous humans, including young children and humans with serious brain damage. … This claim is obviously dangerous for all humans who are weak, vulnerable, and incapacitated.[37]

The defence that Principlism offers to the infant here feels weak. Beauchamp and Childress have not proposed an anthropology of the child that ascribes inherent value to dependence rather than to autonomy. Without it, they have not been able to explain in what the vulnerability of non-autonomous humans might consist. Why, in other words, should it matter how we treat infants? An answer might be that we value the human capacity to depend on others just as highly as we value the capacity for self-rule, but Principlism does not make that response.

Respect for autonomy is one of the pillars of Principlism—some would argue the most important one. Its conception of autonomy was articulated to express the moral freedom of a perfectly rational and perfectly independent person. Beauchamp and Childress' definition shows that they consider that capacity to influence one's environment to be an indispensable component of autonomy. The concept of autonomy considered purely as a capacity for self-rule is, however, adult-normative in principle. It has become so closely identified with the cognitive capacities for reflection, deliberation, and evaluation that are necessary for informed consent that in medical ethics autonomy has come to be considered a normative trait or possession of individual persons, thus excluding children.[38,39] Childness does not equip an individual to be autonomous in that sense and it is hard to see a way in which the infant can manifest autonomy in the way it is currently usually understood in medical ethics. If we want to conclude that a normal infant is autonomous and should not be used 'merely as another's end', we must start to understand autonomy in a different way; one that is within the scope of a human who possesses only the capacities of childness.

---

[36] 'Our obligations to respect autonomy do not extend to persons who cannot act in a sufficiently autonomous manner (and who cannot be rendered autonomous) because they are immature, incapacitated, ignorant, coerced or exploited. Infants, irrationally suicidal individuals and drug-dependent patients are examples' (Ibid., p. 105).

[37] Ibid., p. 72.

[38] Jessica W. Berg, 'The Legal Requirements for Disclosure and Consent: History and Current Status', in Jessica W. Berg and Paul S. Appelbaum (eds.), *Informed consent: legal theory and clinical practice* (2nd edn.; Oxford, New York: Oxford University Press, 2001), 41–74.

[39] Beauchamp and Childress point out that in reality the ability to consent lies on a continuum. Beauchamp and Childress, *Principles of Biomedical Ethics*, pp. 113–17. That idea would potentially enable older children to exercise autonomy as it is understood on adult-normative terms; at least under some circumstances.

5.1.5 Justice as Fairness

There are two broad ways in which justice can be conceived. *Rectificatory* justice describes the idea that each individual should receive what he deserves, while *distributive* justice describes the idea that all people should be treated as equally important. The two are linked by the notion of fairness. In medical ethics, justice as fairness relates primarily to distributive justice.[40] Beauchamp and Childress suggest that it refers to '… fair, equitable and appropriate distribution determined by justified norms that structure the terms of social cooperation … [it] refers broadly to the distribution of all rights and responsibilities in society, including civil and political rights'.[41]

Beauchamp and Childress assert that it is neither possible nor necessary for the form of distributive justice to have its roots in any single moral theory. They set out a number of utilitarian, libertarian, communitarian, egalitarian, and cosmopolitan theories that can reasonably underpin fairness in healthcare and conclude that, although many different theories can contribute usefully to thinking about justice in biomedical ethics, it is consequentialism and John Rawls' egalitarianism that are the two most helpful.[42]

Consequentialism focuses on the doctors' moral responsibility to society. Providing the theoretical need for healthcare costs more than what is available, then distributive justice depends on the consequentialist idea that the moral rightness of a medical ethical decision is in the extent to which it is cost-effective; the extent to which healthcare resources are used in a way that maximises the amount of health

---

[40] Questions of what the individual patient deserves can be important, but they are usually contingent on how healthcare resources are used, which relies on prior understandings of distributive justice. So, for example, Smart argues in 'Fault and the Allocation of Spare Organs' that: '… rectificatory justice should supplement distributive justice in allocating priority of access to scarce medical resources. Where a patient is at fault for the scarcity of healthy organs a principle of restitution requires that she should give priority to the faultless. Such restitution is non-punitive, and is akin to reparation in civil law, not criminal law'. B. Smart, 'Fault and the allocation of spare organs', *J Med Ethics,* 20/1 (Mar 1994), 26–30. It is clear that, if there were no scarcity of organs available for transplant in the first place, the issue of whether or not the patient were at fault would not arise. Similarly, the arguments for giving lower priority to healthcare for patients who are responsible for their own illness do not make any sense unless they are seen in a context in which resources available to pay for that healthcare are constrained: 'The distribution of scarce healthcare resources is an increasingly important issue due to factors such as expensive 'high tech' medicine, longer life expectancies and the rising prevalence of chronic illness. Furthermore, in the current healthcare context lifestyle-related factors such as high blood pressure, tobacco use and obesity are believed to contribute significantly to the global burden of disease … should patients with self-caused illness receive lower priority in access to healthcare resources?' K. Sharkey and L. Gillam, 'Should patients with self-inflicted illness receive lower priority in access to healthcare resources? Mapping out the debate', *J Med Ethics,* 36/11 (Nov 2010), 661–5.

[41] Beauchamp and Childress, *Principles of Biomedical Ethics,* p. 241.

[42] Ibid., p. 280.

that results.[43] Rawls focuses on the responsibility of society to the individual, including its obligation to provide healthcare. The roots of his conception of justice are in the contract tradition of Rousseau and Locke. According to that conception, justice as fairness depends on the persons who comprise society agreeing the various rules by which society is to function, in order that its members are not exploited by one another. Rawls considers society to be an ethical construct, pragmatically designed by its members to achieve the best outcome for the persons who comprise it. A well-ordered society is, he suggests: '… a scheme of cooperation for reciprocal advantage regulated by principles which persons would choose in an initial situation that is fair'.[44] That conception of society relies on Hume's idea that there is, or should be, reciprocity between persons.[45] What a just society should provide to individuals is related to what individual persons should be expected to do for society. Rawls argues that people in society do, in practice, recognise the contribution inequality can make to fairness and are content to accommodate or even to encourage it—but only to the extent that it benefits everyone.[46] Fairness does not necessarily equate with equality. To put it another way, inequality can be fair—but *only* if the 'basic rights and duties' of persons in society are considered to be equal. It is not necessary that the rules should preclude inequality—that might not even be desirable—but it is sine qua non that all members of society contribute to the agreement of those

---

[43] If the only funding available were £1000, and it would either buy a course of antibiotic A for one patient that was 99% likely to work, or provide two patients with a course each of antibiotic B that was 85% likely to work, it would be unfair to spend it all on the more effective antibiotic A, because more health would be achieved with two courses of the less effective antibiotic. If the source of healthcare funding is taxes, then on consequentialist grounds distributive justice expresses that clinicians are morally responsible for ensuring money is spent in a way that benefits as many members of that community as possible; to procure the 'biggest bang for the health-care buck'.

[44] John Rawls, *A Theory of Justice* (Cambridge, MA: Belknap Press of Harvard University Press, 1999), p. 30.

[45] 'All our obligations to do good to society seem to imply something reciprocal. I receive the benefits of society, and therefore ought to promote its interests'. David Hume, *Essays on suicide and the immortality of the soul. By the late David Hume, Esq. With remarks by the editor. To which are added, two letters on suicide, from Rousseau's Eloisa* (A new edn.; Basil: Collection of English Classics, 1799), p. 12.

[46] 'I shall maintain … that the persons in the initial situation would choose two rather different principles: the first requires equality in the assignment of basic rights and duties, while the second holds that social and economic inequalities, for example inequalities of wealth and authority, are just only if they result in compensating benefits for everyone, and in particular for the least advantaged members of society. These principles rule out justifying institutions on the grounds that the hardships of some are offset by a greater good in the aggregate. It may be expedient but it is not just that some should have less in order that others may prosper. *But there is no injustice in the greater benefits earned by a few provided that the situation of persons not so fortunate is thereby improved.* The intuitive idea is that since everyone's well-being depends upon a scheme of cooperation without which no one could have a satisfactory life, the division of advantages should be such as to draw forth the willing cooperation of everyone taking part in it, including those less well situated'. Rawls, *A Theory of Justice*, p. 13 (My italics).

rules, and that such agreement is reached in a way that does not systematically favour some over others.

It is that agreement of the principles of justice, which Rawls calls the 'original position', which defines fairness.[47] The agreement must be reached by correct moral reasoning, which on terms that Rawls agree with Kant means on the basis that everyone participating in the agreement is of equal value. Rawls proposes a device which he calls a 'veil of ignorance' for ensuring such universalisability. Those agreeing the original position know themselves to be free and equal individuals who are of the age of reason, but that is all they know about themselves. They are unaware of their own gender, for example, in order that the rules they agree do not favour males over females. They are unaware of their colour, so that the rules they agree do not favour whites over blacks. They are, in fact, unaware of anything about themselves that might tempt them to prejudice the rules to their own advantage.[48]

The idea can be illustrated by imagining a moral agent walking off a large lunch by strolling down St Giles in Oxford. She might see five identical beggars sitting at intervals along the pavement in front of her, each needing food. There is a sandwich shop at the end of the road, but none of the beggars has any money to buy one. The agent discovers that by chance she has six £1 coins in her pocket. If she were to give one coin to each beggar and keep the remaining one, it would satisfy a strictly consequentialist conception of justice. The universe would approve, because the agent has considered all the beggars' interests equally and the impact on the interests of each of them was the same.

If, however, the cheapest sandwich available to buy actually costs £6.00, the agent's actions have ensured not only that none of the beggars can eat as a result of her decision, but that she herself is no longer in a position to help them. In order to change that state of injustice, she would need to keep all the money to buy a sandwich, and then distribute the sandwich among the five beggars. It is an illustration of Aristotle's articulation that a principle of formal equality demands not only that 'equals should be treated equally' but also that 'unequals should be treated unequally'.[49] In other words, inequality can paradoxically serve the ends of justice, while equality can frustrate them.

But only if the reasons for that inequality are reasonable. Each of the beggars might reasonably feel peeved as the agent simply walked past without disbursing a coin, but if she set out her plan beforehand and—critically—explained its reasoning, it is likely they would agree that there was a sense in which it was a fair plan; the only plan, moreover, that would result in each of them becoming less hungry. In

---

[47] '… the guiding idea is that the principles of justice for the basic structure of society are the object of the original agreement. They are the principles that free and rational persons concerned to further their own interests would accept in an initial position of equality as defining the fundamental terms of their association. These principles are to regulate all further agreements; they specify the kinds of social cooperation that can be entered into and the forms of government that can be established' (Ibid., p. 10).

[48] Ibid., p. 221.

[49] Beauchamp and Childress, *Principles of Biomedical Ethics*, p. 242.

order for the plan to be fair, there must be an initial agreement between the beggar and the agent that she can keep all the money, on the understanding that she will spend it on a sandwich which she will then share equally between herself and the five beggars. It is that agreement, as well as in operation of the principles that result from the agreement, that ensures societal justice is served.

5.1.6 *Justice and Childness*

A concept of society as a community of reciprocating moral agents leads quickly to a distinctly adult-normative definition of personal value. Tristram Engelhardt Jr. considers that it is societal reciprocity that provides us with a definition of a person 'in the strict sense'.[50] A person, on those terms, is someone who can reasonably be held accountable by others for what he has done and is able to hold himself accountable for what he does. To be considered a member of the community of persons on those terms, an individual must be capable of moral agency.[51] On those grounds, the status of children and infants is far from clear. They are not persons, at least in the strict sense to which Engelhardt refers, because in the present moment they do not participate in society in the way that a rational adult would, so it is not clear in what sense they can cooperate to reciprocal advantage.

Beauchamp and Childress find a place for infants and children in society by drawing a distinction between those who are moral actors and those who are part of a moral community. The child or infant is not yet a moral actor. Along with companion animals, infants and children do, however, merit a place in society if it is considered as a moral community, albeit only as a sort of apprentice who is learning the trade, a potential moral actor.[52] Drawing on Rawls, Principlism considers society to be: '… determined by justified norms that structure the terms of social cooperation'.[53] Fairness, on those terms, can consist partly in society's maintaining a system ('norms') in which some patients are treated differently from others. Justice-as-fairness is not served solely by equality. It is not served, for example, if a doctor decides to intervene in the same way for every patient without considering the

---

[50] 'One speaks of persons in order to identify entities one can with warrant blame or praise, which can themselves blame or praise, and which can as a result play a role in the core of the moral life. In order to engage in moral discourse, such entities will need to reflect on themselves; they must therefore be self- conscious. They will need to be rational beings. That rationality must include an understanding of the notion of worthiness of blame and praise: a minimal moral sense' (Engelhardt, *The Foundations of Bioethics*, p. 139).

[51] See also Ibid., p. 156.

[52] '… many individuals into the moral community that are not moral actors in that community. Babies and companion animals are examples. This theory tries to capture the conditions under which certain relationships, especially those involving social interaction and reciprocity, are stronger and more influential than relationships with strangers and others outside an interpersonal connection'. Beauchamp and Childress, *Principles of Biomedical Ethics*, p. 79.

[53] Ibid., p. 241.

extent to which the patient can benefit or will be harmed by it. Society can serve justice by agreeing a material principle that maintains inequality.[54]

When it comes to infants and children, the keyword here is 'justified'. In order for the structure of social cooperation to be fair, equitable and appropriate, the norms that structure the terms of it must be rationally explained. If a doctor treats one patient differently from another, the reason for that difference must not be arbitrary; it must be explainable by something that makes the two persons distinct in a way that is relevant to that moral decision. Unequal treatment is fair only to the extent that characteristics of individuals can explain such inequality. A fair healthcare system permits different access to resources based on gender, for example, but only to the extent that the difference is relevant to the resource in question. It is reasonable to offer mammograms to women but not men because there is an objective difference between women and men that is relevant. It would not be reasonable if the reason were simply that society valued women more highly.

Society has certainly agreed that infants and children can be treated differently from adults. We allow parents to influence medical decision-making over children in ways that would be unthinkable if the patient were an adult. Adult-normativity represents a societal norm and, like other societal norms, in order to accord with Beauchamp and Childress' principle of justice, it is only fair if it can be justified. An ethical account that treats normal infants and adults differently is fair to the extent that it can show convincingly that there are inherent characteristics that explain the basis for such unequal treatment.

The explanation that Rawls offers is only partial. Infants and children are not 'of the age of reason' and, as we have seen, are excluded from those agreeing the original position.[55] Although one of Rawls' objectives is to show that utilitarian consequentialism is a flawed basis for justice, in respect of infants and children his egalitarian theory reaches many of the same conclusions that consequentialism does. Both consider society to be a community of moral persons, making it necessary to reach an agreed definition of who is in that community. The effect of both is to make a faculty for moral reasoning (and therefore calculative logic) the sine qua non for that definition, and both conclude that childness changes the moral value of

---

[54] Thus, when the parent of a cognitively impaired child expresses to the paediatrician that 'What I need to know is that you will treat my child exactly as you would any other child', she does not expect that the paediatrician will ignore her child's disabilities in making treatment decisions. Rather, she expects that the rational and compassionate paediatrician will only take disabilities into account to the extent that they are relevant because they impact rationally on the extent to which the harms of an intervention are justified by its benefits.

[55] 'The child has not yet mastered the art of perceiving the person of others, that is, the art of discerning their beliefs, intentions, and feelings, so that an awareness of these things cannot inform his interpretation of their behavior. Moreover, his ability to put himself in their place is still untutored and likely to lead him astray. It is no surprise, then, that these elements, so important from the final moral point of view, are left out of account at the earliest stage ...' Rawls, *A Theory of Justice*, p. 411.

an individual when it comes to justice as fairness.[56] Both offer attempts to justify that difference on the adult-normative grounds that childness—the infant's appreciation and awareness of the universe—is less valid for moral status than that of the ideal adult.

Rawls is nevertheless able to accommodate a meaningful role for infants in his account of justice, but only because one of the agreements reached by those in the original position is that the vulnerable are cared for in a way that cannot be justified on the basis of reciprocity alone. The child exemplifies the sort of irrationality against which the parties to the original position protect themselves by agreeing to the non-ideal, but necessary, principle of paternalism as a 'protection against our own irrationality'.[57] A paternalistic decision flows from what is objectively and rationally 'good for' the child, according to the thin conception of the good that is represented by the original position (as well as from the child's own wishes to the extent that they are rational).[58]

According to this non-ideal theory, then, the principle of justice in relation to children consists both in soliciting and acting on preferences that can be expressed and are rational, and in making decisions that are objectively good for the child. It is to Rawls' device of the 'non-ideal' that Principlism appeals in seeking to explain the value of infants and children; an acknowledgement that there are ways in which society as a practical construct differs from what might be considered perfect from a purely rational and hypothetical perspective. One of the ways in which society differs from the ideal, according to Beauchamp and Childress, is that society should in practice give value to some human beings who cannot participate in reciprocity.

That protects infants but, again, only by virtue of considering them an exception to a more general rule derived from what should obtain in adults. Individuals who demonstrate childness are accommodated only by the non-ideal theory of

---

[56] For some bioethicists, that difference extends to a belief that infants can be extinguished without injustice. For Rawls, it means the onus of justice as fairness is on the family, rather than on society. Although the two claims of value are wildly different, neither allows the infant full status as a person on grounds that are adult-normative. See also Stephen R. L. Clark, *The political animal: biology, ethics, and politics* (London, New York: Routledge, 2001), p. 59. 'That children below "the age of reason" have no rights in their own right is a necessary consequence of any doctrine that limits the class of rights holders to the class of recognisably and actually rational entities, entities whose deliberate co-operation is needed if any corporate action is to be undertaken, and whose forbearance can only be purchased by reciprocal forbearance'.

[57] '…once the ideal conception is chosen, [parties in the original position] will want to insure themselves against the possibility that their powers are undeveloped and they cannot rationally advance their interests, as in the case of children. For these cases the parties adopt principles stipulating when others are authorized to act in their behalf and to override their present wishes if necessary; and this they do recognizing that sometimes their capacity to act rationally for their good may fail, or be lacking altogether'. (Rawls, *A Theory of Justice*, pp. 218–20.) See also Beauchamp and Childress, *Principles of Biomedical Ethics*, pp. 209–10.

[58] 'Paternalistic decisions are to be guided by the individual's own settled preferences and interests insofar as they are not irrational, or failing a knowledge of these, by the theory of primary goods. As we know less and less about a person, we act for him as we would act for ourselves from the standpoint of the original position' (Rawls, *A Theory of Justice*, pp. 218–20).

paternalism. The value of infants and children once again seems to flow, not from their own inherent childness, but from the obligations that adultness imposes on adults. The challenge that offers to an adult-normative account of what sorts of human beings need not be treated fairly by human society is weak.

5.2 Summary

Principlism sets out a series of obligations to patients that medical ethics imposes on healthcare professionals. Its principles are an obligation to further a patient's interests, both by avoiding harm and by actively causing benefit, an obligation to respect autonomy and an obligation to act fairly in accordance with conceptions of justice.

Explaining why those obligations should extend to infants and children is not straightforward. Principlism's most strident assertion is that the source of a duty to concern oneself with the interests of a child is the nature of the agent's relationship with him. That account of duty and relationship is attractive because it gives a value to the life of an infant that is not exhausted by the consequentialist impact that the infant has on others. But it does not succeed in refuting a fundamental consequentialist claim that an infant's appreciation of her existence does not amount to a capacity to have interests, because the central idea of relationship on which it relies is ambiguous. Beauchamp and Childress indicate that the relationships they are talking about are defined by the obligations which parties in that relationship should expect. Children should expect adults to care for them, especially when those adults are the child's parents. But that means the relationship simultaneously defines and is defined by those obligations. The reasoning appears circular; a morally relevant relationship is defined as one which imposes obligations, while a moral agent's obligations are defined by her relationship with the moral 'patient'. The agent's relationship with an individual is defined by the duties she takes on, while at the same time the relationship determines the obligations that such a duty represents. It is not clear in Principlism which comes first. There are points at which the source of value is considered to be prior to that of duty, and others at which duty is seen to be prior to value.

Principlism's deontological account of the child's inherent value does not, in summary, appeal to anything that is objectively true about the child's inherent value, and so seems to be trying to pick itself up by its own bootstraps. Whichever direction the arrow of causality goes—whether from duty to value or from value to duty—Principlism relies on axiomatic assumptions about the way idealised rational beings 'ought' to consider infants and children, that are ultimately drawn simply from the way in which people currently *do* consider them. The fact that virtually everyone agrees on something does not mean that they will always agree, or that they are right in any rational sense to do so.

Principlism's second obligation is to respect autonomy. Contemporary understanding of autonomy requires the individual person to have an adult ability to give informed consent to interventions, which relies on specific reasoning that infants do not possess. Principlism rejects the conclusion that the moral agent can value non-autonomous humans less highly than humans who possess autonomy. The grounds for that rejection are that the obligation to respect autonomy does not flow from the nature of the moral patient at all, but from the nature of the moral agent and his relationship with the moral patient. But, without proposing an alternative account of autonomy that is not dependent on the characteristics of adultness, it is not clear what demands such an obligation might make in respect of infants and children. On the terms that Principlism sets out, the evaluative power of autonomy is that it represents the capacities that permit self-rule. An individual is exploited if she possesses those capacities but is denied the opportunity to use them and instead is used merely as a 'means to another's end'. Beauchamp and Childress note that it is intuitively repugnant to allow adults to treat infants merely as objects, but the concept of autonomy that they present does not provide an explanation as to why that repugnance is morally justified. Since childness does not encompass the capacities necessary for self-rule, the principle of respect for autonomy does not apply. On the basis of Principlism's understanding of autonomy as self-rule, it is not clear in what way an infant can be exploited.

The final duty in Principlism is justice. Principlism considers society to be a community of moral persons. The moral question then becomes who should be included in that community and what criteria should define its membership. Principlism insists that infants and children have a place in the moral community, but on contractarian terms it is not clear what that place should be. The fact that someone will probably develop a capacity to reciprocate in the future does not obviously constitute a reason for treating her as though she were already a member of society now. Part of the 'original position', taken behind Rawls' veil of ignorance, is that a fair society will treat infants as persons, even though the infant is unable to reciprocate morally in the present moment. But it is not clear why rational people should make such an agreement, since even behind the veil of ignorance they are allowed the knowledge that they are not infants. Despite Rawls' fundamental objections to consequentialism, the alternative he sets out, and on which Principlism draws, makes adultness the touchstone for membership of a moral community in much the same way that consequentialism does. Both theories justify societal norms that value childness less highly than adultness and therefore represent a specifically adult-normative conception of justice—one that excludes those who are not rational in the adult sense for no better reason than that it is not the way adults reason. In that case, there seems no obvious way in which a being who does not reason like an adult can be included in the community of moral actor-patients.

The diverse range of moral theories on which Principlism draws has meant it has been able to provide infants and children with considerable protection over the decades since it first appeared. Principlism's authors consistently affirm the inherent value of infants and children, but the moral reasoning behind that affirmation is not always clear or persuasive because it does not rely on anything that is inherently or objectively true about infants or children themselves. Instead, it evaluates children with reference to what is true about adults, such as the nature of adults' proper relationship with children, or agreements between adults about the obligations that such relationships impose on adults, or how adults should deal with individuals who don't quite make the grade yet as humans with full value. It does not challenge the fundamental idea that ultimately it is only the characteristics of adultness that can confer full inherent personal value on an individual. What Principlism and the moral theories on which it draws have failed to do, in other words, is to call into question adult-normativity itself.

Bibliography

Baines P. Medical ethics for children: applying the four principles to paediatrics. J Med Ethics. 2008;34(3):141–5.

Beauchamp TL. Principlism and its alleged competitors. Kennedy Inst Ethics J. 1995;5(3):181–98.

Beauchamp T, Childress J. Principles of biomedical ethics. 6th ed. New York: Oxford University Press; 2009.

Berg JW. The legal requirements for disclosure and consent: history and current status. In: Berg JW, Appelbaum PS, editors. Informed consent: legal theory and clinical practice. 2nd ed. Oxford/New York: Oxford University Press; 2001. p. 41–74.

Berlin I. Two concepts of liberty: an inaugural lecture delivered before the University of Oxford on 31 October 1958. Oxford: Clarendon Press; 1958.

Childress JF. Protestant perspectives on informed consent (particularly in research involving human participants). Fordham Urban Law J. 2002;30(1 art 11):187–205.

Clark SRL. The political animal: biology, ethics, and politics. London/New York: Routledge; 2001.

Echteld MA, et al. Quality of life change and response shift in patients admitted to palliative care units: a pilot study. Palliat Med. 2005;19(5):381–8.

Echteld MA, et al. Changes in and correlates of individual quality of life in advanced cancer patients admitted to an academic unit for palliative care. Palliat Med. 2007;21(3):199–205.

Engelhardt HT. The foundations of bioethics. New York: Oxford University Press; 1996.

General Medical Council. Good medical practice. London: General Medical Council; 2023.

Green B. Use of the Hippocratic or other professional oaths in UK medical schools in 2017: practice, perception of benefit and principlism. BMC Res Notes. 2017;10(1):777.

Hume D. Essays on suicide and the immortality of the soul. By the late David Hume, Esq. With remarks by the editor. To which are added, two letters on suicide, from Rousseau's Eloisa. A new ed. Basil: Collection of English Classics; 1799.

Kant I, Wood AW, Schneewind JB. Groundwork for the metaphysics of morals, Rethinking the Western tradition. New Haven: Yale University Press; 2002.

Mill JS. Chapter V. Applications. In: Courtney WL, editor. On liberty. London and Felling-on-Tyne, New York and Melbourne: The Walter Scott Publishing Co., Ltd.; 1901.

O'Neill O. Autonomy and trust in bioethics, Gifford lectures. Cambridge: Cambridge University Press; 2002.

Rachels J. Can ethics provide answers? And other essays in moral philosophy. Lanham/London: Rowman & Littlefield; 1997.

Ramsey P. The enforcement of morals: nontherapeutic research on children. Hast Cent Rep. 1976;6(4):21–30.

Ramsey P. The patient as person: explorations in medical ethics. Yale University Press; 2002.
Rawls J. A theory of justice. Cambridge, MA: Belknap Press of Harvard University Press; 1999.
Schapiro T. What is a child? Ethics. 1999;109(4):715–38.
Sharkey K, Gillam L. Should patients with self-inflicted illness receive lower priority in access to healthcare resources? Mapping out the debate. J Med Ethics. 2010;36(11):661–5.
Singer P. Famine, affluence and morality. Philos Public Aff. 1972;1(1):229–43.
Singer P. Practical ethics. New York: Cambridge University Press; 2011.
Smart B. Fault and the allocation of spare organs. J Med Ethics. 1994;20(1):26–30.

Chapter 6
Childness in Consequentialism

6.1 Consequentialism 101

An ideal moral theory would describe a way of evaluating moral action that sets aside individual issues of personal perspective or metaphysical worldview so that it can explain an action's 'rightness' in a way that is true for everyone, always and everywhere. Consequentialist moral theories aim to achieve that by establishing a unit of value that is so fundamental that everyone can—or should—agree on the value it indicates. That something, according to consequentialist moral theories, is the outcome of an agent's action.

Consequentialists do not have to agree on what that outcome should be. Libertarian consequentialists might argue that the measure of an action's 'rightness' is the extent to which it increases the universe's store of freedom among human beings. Classical utilitarian consequentialists would suggest that an action is right to the extent to which it increases the universe's store of happiness or reduces its suffering, while some preference utilitarians equate 'rightness' with the extent to which personal preferences are globally maximised. What consequentialist theories have in common is that their focus is on practical outcomes, rather than, for example, the agent's disposition or willingness to adhere to a certain moral code. Concerns other than outcome might be relevant to ethical deliberation, but ultimately that relevance is only to the extent that they impact the consequences of any action the moral agent might take. The value of a doctor's intention, for example, can be expressed in more fundamental terms as the moral value of the consequences she expects to result from her actions. According to most consequentialist thinking, numinous ethical concepts such as virtue, dignity or honour are not valuable in themselves, although they too might be relevant to the extent that they influence the overall impact of an

R. Hain, *Childness and the Myth of the Unfinished Human*,
https://doi.org/10.1007/978-3-032-12111-0_6

agent's action.[1] Most moral theories, consequentialist or otherwise, recognise that the outcome of an action is relevant to its moral value; what is distinctive about consequentialism is its claim that the outcome is ultimately *all* that matters. A great deal, therefore, hangs on what the desirable outcome of moral action is taken to be.

Many philosophers have identified structural weaknesses in the logic of consequentialism. Moral philosopher Bernard Williams points out that consequentialist theories explain what should be done by somebody (what Williams describes as 'the state of affairs'), but consequentialism fails to explain why it is the obligation of the individual agent to do it and so does not obviously guide an individual moral agent's action.[2] There is little moral difference on consequentialist grounds between an agent's failure to attend to the needs of the person immediately in front of her, and her failure to attend to the needs of everyone else, at all times and in all places.[3] At the very moment the agent is acting morally correctly in respect of one individual, and indeed in the same action, he is therefore technically considered by consequentialism to be acting wrongly in respect of everyone else. The task of acting correctly thereby becomes impossible, so that it can be argued that most forms of consequentialism effectively decouple the moral value of a decision from an agent's moral reasoning. Williams expressed the hope in 1963 that 'The day cannot be too far off when we hear no more of [utilitarian consequentialism]'.[4]

Despite Williams' misgivings, consequentialism has survived. In medical ethics, it has even flourished, because it is in many ways an attractive moral philosophy for clinicians. Consequentialism is good at expressing moral ideas in terms that clinicians recognise are relevant to their everyday practice of medicine. It asserts that ethics has a purpose and that the goal of ethics, like that of medicine itself, is to improve the quality of humans' existence. It is practical and makes few metaphysical demands on the conscientious clinician. By ethically evaluating an action in terms of its impact on a patient, consequentialism even holds out the promise that moral rightness and wrongness can become measurable in the same way that the effectiveness of a medical intervention is usually measurable.[5] Making moral

---

[1] Peter Singer, for example, discounts the concept of 'dignity' in ethical debate on the grounds that it is intangible. ('We all know what preferences are, whereas claims that something is intrinsically morally wrong, or violates a natural right, or is contrary to human dignity invoke less tangible concepts that make their truth more difficult to assess.') Singer, *Practical Ethics*, p. 51.

[2] Bernard Arthur Owen Williams, 'A critique of utilitarianism', in J. J. C Smart and Bernard Arthur Owen Williams (eds.), *Utilitarianism: for and against* (Cambridge: Cambridge University Press, 1987), p. 93.

[3] '… because consequentialism attaches value ultimately to states of affairs the world contains, … it essentially involves the notion of *negative responsibility*: that if I am ever responsible for anything, then I must be just as much responsible for things that I allow or fail to prevent, as I am for things that I myself, in the more everyday restricted sense, bring about' (Ibid., p. 95).

[4] Ibid., p. 150.

[5] The drive for an approach to medical ethics that is practical means that healthcare sciences are particularly prone to give inappropriate weight to outcomes that are measurable, rather than those that are meaningful. See D. Swinglehurst et al., 'Confronting the quality paradox: towards new characterisations of 'quality' in contemporary healthcare', *BMC Health Services Research,* 15/1 (2015) 3.

decisions can, hypothetically, become as straightforward as establishing a dose–response curve in pharmacology and therapeutics. Where other moral theories complicate medical decisions by introducing ideas of virtue and duty that might be in tension with what is expedient, consequentialism presents clinicians with the seductive possibility that what is morally correct in principle might always align itself with what is clinically convenient in practice. Some forms of consequentialism can, for example, claim with some confidence to identify certain human beings who lack the capacity to suffer from or benefit from medical or other interventions, and who, in consequentialist terms, therefore lack any personal value at all. Such individuals, it is suggested, are not truly persons and can be despatched without moral qualm. That would resolve many of the complex moral quandaries in which healthcare professionals currently find themselves, particularly in the face of increasingly competitive healthcare resources.

The practical utility of consequentialist theories stands in their favour as a basis for reasoning in medical ethics (though it should also make them somewhat alarming; clinicians should perhaps be wary of any moral theory that identifies virtue quite so closely with pragmatism). Few would dispute the idea that outcome matters morally in clinical practice. Most of the moral theories from which medical ethics is derived are based ultimately on some formulation of the golden rule, 'Treat others as you would want to be treated', which entails that there is a connection between the sort of action an agent is morally obliged to take and the outcome that is expected to result. Most of the time, ethical medical decision-making relies largely on knowing what the effects of an intervention are likely to be, and only proceeding if its benefits are likely to exceed its harms. Ethical reasoning about an intervention cannot simply be a matter of deciding what code or codes are relevant and working out how to adhere to them. Whether or not Williams is right to be sceptical about it as a comprehensive and coherent moral theory, some form of consequentialism seems to have a place in practical medical ethics. Consequentialism may be wrong to claim that consequences are *all* that matter morally, but in medical ethics it seems reasonable to accept that consequences are at least prominent *among* the things that matter.

6.2   The Vulnerability of Infants and Children

Several factors combine to mean that consequentialism is more prone than other ethical theories to the prejudicial effects of adult-normative thinking. Unlike bioethical approaches that are based on ideas of duty or disposition, consequentialist theories connect the value of a person to what that person is like. A key claim of consequentialism is that the moral agent's obligations to an individual extend only as far as that individual's capacity to benefit from an action the agent might take. Consequentialist theories link an individual's value firmly to her ability to benefit from (or be harmed by) moral action. That represents personal value exclusively as a function (in the mathematical sense) of an individual's abilities, which, if they are evaluated with reference to what is normal for adults, introduces bias and systematically under-expresses the value of infants and children. That locates the patient's inherent value in the capacities he possesses that permit him so to benefit. Consequentialism connects the extent to which the agent should concern himself with an individual's interests to that individual's capacity to participate in the desirable outcome preferred by the consequentialist theory in question.

An analogy might be to consider a landlord who owns a flat. As a landlord, he is bound by regulations in the *Landlord's Book of Rules*. Among those regulations is a clause that says landlords must maintain the décor of the flat, making sure it is attractive to the tenants. One day there is a surprise inspection and the inspector notes that the landlord has painted the flat using cheap grey paint instead of expensive coloured paint. When asked why, the landlord explains that his current tenants are colour-blind. On utilitarian consequentialist grounds, the landlord has acted perfectly correctly, because it does not matter to the tenants what colour the walls are and the money the landlord saves by using cheap grey paint can (presumably) be used in some other way to increase the sum total of human happiness. The moral rightness of the landlord's action is determined, in other words, by characteristics of the beneficiaries of his action, and not just by his own disposition, or by any obligations he might have.

In utilitarian consequentialist terms, an individual's value—considered as the extent to which a moral agent should concern herself with that individual's interests—is an expression of that individual's capacity to suffer or be made happy. At one end of the spectrum, a stone has no interests with which the moral agent need concern herself. A mouse, in contrast, is capable of suffering at the hands of the moral agent and so the moral agent has a moral obligation to avoid inflicting such suffering.[6] Most adult human beings, with their complex capacity for existential as well as physical suffering, lie at the other end of the capacity-to-suffer spectrum and so the moral agent's obligation to avoid inflicting suffering on adult human beings is correspondingly great.

---

[6]As Singer explains: 'It would be nonsense to say that it was not in the interests of a stone to be kicked along the road by a child. A stone does not have interests because it cannot suffer. Nothing that we can do to it could possibly make any difference to its welfare. A mouse, on the other hand, does have an interest in not being tormented, because mice will suffer if they are treated in this way'. Singer, *Practical Ethics*, p. 50.

6.2.1   Zero-Setting

Consequentialist theories find it disconcertingly easy to set an individual's personal value at zero without reference to any standard that is external to the theory itself. The connection which consequentialism makes between the rightness of a moral action and the capacities of the beneficiary of that action means that consequentialist theoreticians are easily convinced about the sort of patient whose interests need not concern the doctor. Consequentialist theories that explain personal value are often distinguished by a willingness to draw confident conclusions about who or what entirely *lacks* that value; a willingness that extends beyond philosophical abstractions and permits consequentialism to set at zero the value of extant individuals who lack certain capacities. Consequentialist theories are typically comfortable with the idea that there are human beings who do not 'count' in the moral calculus because, on consequentialist grounds, there is no moral obligation on the agent to concern herself with the interests of someone who cannot benefit from ethically correct behaviour.[7] Exactly which capacities matter depends on the moral task that a specific theory has set itself. An ability to perceive colour is only valuable to the extent that the desirable outcome depends on perceiving colour. To a hedonistic utilitarian, the capacities that matter are those that permit the individual to experience pleasure or suffering and be aware of that experience, while to a preference utilitarian they are the capacities needed to formulate a preference.

Clinicians talk about two ways in which a laboratory test might be inaccurate. One is that a test gives a false positive when in fact everything is normal. The other is that the it is falsely negative when in fact there is a problem. When it comes to ascribing personal value, consequentialist theories are unlikely to give a false positive. To pursue the earlier metaphor, the explanation that consequentialism provides as to why it is important to keep an apartment attractive when its tenants *can* perceive colour is compelling. If the tenants in an apartment have normal colour vision, then their capacity to experience colour is an excellent reason for painting it colourfully. But it does not follow logically that consequentialism is equally right to claim that if tenants are colour-blind there is no need for such attention. Deontologists might insist that the landlord has an obligation to maintain the flat in a way that is attractive to most people because, in becoming a landlord, he has made himself subordinate to the regulations set out in the *Landlord's Book of Rules*. Virtue ethicists might point out that a good landlord would always want to do the best for his tenants anyway, whether they themselves are aware of it or not.

Consequentialist theories are likely to be correct where they *do* ascribe value to a person, but is at risk of *failing* to ascribe value where, in fact, such personal value exists.[8] If a theory considers an individual to possess inherent value only to the

---

[7] Jeremy Bentham, *An introduction to the principles of morals and legislation* (Principles of morals and legislation; Oxford: Clarendon Press, 1879), p. 311.

[8] S. Holm, 'The peaceable pluralistic society and the question of persons', *J Med Philos,* 13/4 (Nov 1988), 379–86.

extent that he can participate in the desirable outcome, and then defines the desirable outcome in a way that does not represent all the ways in which humans can enjoy their existence, the value it returns will be a false negative. That is, the theory will reject as irrelevant capacities that, in reality, do equip a person to be able to enjoy their existence.[9] It is quite easy to make a false start in consequentialism by a wrong judgement about what the desirable outcome should be.

The more broadly a consequentialist theory conceives of the desirable outcome, the less that risk becomes. To avoid false negatives, a consequentialist ethical theory must have as its objective an outcome that is sufficiently broad to accord value to the myriad different ways in which people in the real world can flourish. If we define the desirable outcome broadly enough, we can start to see consequentialist reasons why a landlord should keep the flat colourful even if his tenants cannot appreciate it. The tenants, unable to perceive colour themselves, might derive benefit from the pleasure their colour-aware dinner guests can obtain from a colourfully painted apartment. Behaving honourably might promote the landlord's own well-being.

In his classical formulation of utilitarian consequentialism, Bentham reduces human flourishing to a single scale with happiness at one end and suffering at the other.[10] The quality of an individual's existence, he suggests, can be expressed simply as 'happiness' and it is the opposite of suffering, in the same way that a negative number is the opposite of a positive one.[11] Indeed, in its purest form, utilitarian consequentialism sees moral reasoning as an exercise in arithmetic, in which the agent arrives at a decision by subtracting the amount of suffering from the amount of happiness it will cause. The classical utilitarian use of the term 'happiness' to mean merely pleasure and/or the absence of suffering is difficult to defend. It stands in marked contrast, for example, with its much broader meaning when 'happiness' is used to represent an approximate translation of what Aristotle means by

---

[9] There is, moreover, a sort of philosophical 'blind spot' in consequentialism. Once a consequentialist theory is committed to a certain desirable outcome, it is not only unable to recognise value that does not connect to that outcome; it is unaware that such a lacuna exists N. Agar, 'How to insure against utilitarian overconfidence', *Monash Bioeth Rev,* 32/3–4 (Sep–Dec 2014), 162–71.

[10] "The French have already discovered that the blackness of the skin is no reason why a human being should be abandoned without redress to the caprice of a tormentor. It may 1 day come to be recognised that the number of the legs, the villosity of the skin, or the termination of the os sacrum, are reasons equally insufficient for abandoning a sensitive being to the same fate. What else is it that should trace the insuperable line? Is it the faculty of reason, or perhaps the faculty of discourse? … The question is not, Can they reason? Nor Can they talk? but, Can they suffer? "Bentham, *An introduction to the principles of morals and legislation,* p. 311.

[11] "… the masses and sophisticated people call it happiness, understanding being happy as equivalent to living well and acting well [but] they disagree about substantive conceptions of happiness, the masses giving an account which differs from that of the philosophers. For the masses think it is something straightforward and obvious, like pleasure, wealth, or honour, some thinking it to be one thing, others another." Aristotle, *Nicomachean ethics,* trans. Roger Crisp (Cambridge texts in the history of philosophy; Cambridge: Cambridge University Press, 2000), pp. 4–5 (1095a).

eudaimonia.[12] In the real world, suffering, as well as happiness, can paradoxically contribute to flourishing.

The history of utilitarianism has largely been one of retreat from Bentham's reductionist position.[13] Mill introduced the idea that there is a sense in which some forms of happiness are better than others because they are experienced by beings with more wisdom. That difference is morally relevant, he suggests, because an understanding of higher pleasures enriches lives even when the pleasures themselves are not satisfied.[14] Henry Sidgwick elaborated and explained that difference by drawing a curious distinction between the experience of being happy (or suffering) and the awareness that one is being happy or suffering.[15] A pig can be happy,

---

[12] John Stuart Mill, *A system of logic, ratiocinative and inductive: being a connected view of the principles of evidence and the methods of scientific investigation* (Peoples edn.; London: Longmans, Green, Reader, and Dyer, 1884), p. 175.

[13] There may be a medical explanation for Bentham's narrow conception of human well-being. It is highly likely that he suffered from a condition which was unrecognised at the time but would later be called Asperger's Syndrome and, later still, Autistic Spectrum Disorder (Lucas, P. and Sheeran, A. (2006), 'Asperger's Syndrome and the Eccentricity and Genius of Jeremy Bentham', *Journal of Bentham Studies*, 8, 1–37.) Individuals with Asperger's have a normal, or sometimes unusually acute, faculty for logic. They find it difficult, however, to comprehend anything that is not observable in itself or else can be directly deduced from what is observed. Individuals with Asperger's understand the meaning of the words contained in a phrase that is said to them, for example, but cannot always infer anything from the tone in which it is said or the facial expression which accompanies it about what someone is feeling. A philosophy such as Bentham's extreme form of utilitarianism, that isolates happiness as an abstraction from the lived existence of actual people, is exactly what one would expect from someone with Asperger's who wanted good things for people but found people themselves an impenetrable mystery. While applauding the principles underlying Bentham's moral theory, Mill had little liking for Bentham himself. He believed Bentham lacked compassion and neither had insight into the fact that he lacked it nor recognised that others possessed it, so that he failed to recognise the '… incompleteness of his own mind as a representative of universal human nature. In many of the most natural and strongest feelings of human nature he had no sympathy; from many of its graver experiences he was altogether cut off; and the faculty by which one mind understands a mind different from itself, and throws itself into the feelings of that other mind, was denied him by his deficiency of Imagination' (Mill, J.S. (1859), *Dissertations and Discussions: Political, Philosophical and Historical*, 2 vols. (1; London: John W. Parker and Son), 353). That deficiency led Bentham, in Mill's view, to be too cynical in his stark representation of individual motivation as irredeemably selfish. Today, there is evidence that utilitarian solutions to moral dilemmas are more likely among those with damage to certain parts of the brain (M. Koenigs et al., 'Damage to the prefrontal cortex increases utilitarian moral judgements', *Nature*, 446/7138 (Apr 19 2007), 908–11).

[14] 'It is indisputable that the being whose capacities of enjoyment are low, has the greatest chance of having them fully satisfied; and a highly-endowed being will always feel that any happiness which he can look for, as the world is constituted, is imperfect. But … It is better to be a human being dissatisfied than a pig satisfied; better to be Socrates dissatisfied than a fool satisfied. And if the fool, or the pig, is of a different opinion, it is because they only know their own side of the question. The other party to the comparison knows both sides' (John Stuart Mill, *Utilitarianism* (London: Longmans, Green and Co., 1879), pp. 25–30).

[15] Sidgwick distances himself from Bentham's premise that pleasure itself is the only intrinsic good. It is, he says, the '… desirable *consciousness* which we must regard as ultimate good' (Henry Sidgwick, *The complete works and select correspondence of Henry Sidgwick* (Sidgwick, complete works and select correspondence; Charlottesville, Va.: InteLex Corporation, 1996), p. 397.). My italics.

but in contrast with most humans, a pig is unaware that happiness is, as it were, happening to it. Despite such attempts to preserve the seductive simplicity and universality at the heart of Bentham's proposition without capitulating to the latter's somewhat claustrophobic conception of humans and their happiness, a tradition of reductionism has continued into consequentialist bioethics in the twentieth century. Hedonistic utilitarian consequentialist bioethicist Helga Kuhse, for example, rejects the whole idea of the sanctity of life in medicine and wishes to express personal value exclusively in terms of capacities that allow their possessor to enjoy what Kuhse considers to be a life with quality. Following Sidgwick, she starts '… with the assumption that conscious life has value because it enables the existence of pleasurable states of consciousness'.[16] 'What I am suggesting, then', she goes on, 'is that there is a strong connection between the value of life and the interests of the being whose life it is'.[17] That must be true as far as it goes, but Kuhse does not stop at arguing that there is a strong connection between them. She asserts that interests are *only* expressible as 'pleasurable states of consciousness'. Kuhse is right that the life of a person who is enjoying her existence has value, and that her enjoyment is part of the explanation for it. But while the value of her life cannot be *less* than what is conferred by her enjoyment of it, there is no logical reason why its value might not be *more* than what can be explained by that alone. The quality of an individual's existence is not reducible to that one emotional response. An experience can be painful or upsetting and yet be meaningful and even, in the end, contribute to someone's well-being.

Most of the consequentialist theories that have informed contemporary medical ethics in infants and children have defined personal value in ways that are both narrow and adult-normative. Preference utilitarian Peter Singer, for example, links it to a capacity to formulate and hold meaningful preferences, while John Harris asserts that personal value is merely a function of a capacity for autonomy.[18] Most modern consequentialist understanding of childness can be traced to Michael Tooley's 1972 essay *Abortion and Infanticide*.[19] Tooley's target is the idea that human beings have

---

[16] Helga Kuhse, *The sanctity-of-life doctrine in medicine: a critique* (Oxford: Clarendon Press, 1987), 213.

[17] Ibid., p. 214.

[18] Helga Kuhse, *The sanctity-of-life doctrine in medicine: a critique* (Oxford: Clarendon Press, 1987). See also Harris John Harris, 'Euthanasia and the value of life', in John Keown (ed.), *Euthanasia Examined: Ethical, Clinical and Legal Perspectives* (Cambridge: Cambridge University Press, 1995), p. 11. For critiques of Singer's articulation of preference utilitarianism, see A. Sloane, 'Singer, preference utilitarianism and infanticide', *Stud Christ Ethics,* 12/2 (1999), 47–73, T. A. Long, 'Two philosophers in search of a contradiction: a response to Singer and Kuhse', *J Med Ethics,* 16/2 (Jun 1990), 95–6, Camosy, 'Engaging with Peter Singer', in *God, the good, and utilitarianism: perspectives on Peter Singer*, Susan F. Krantz, *Refuting Peter Singer's ethical theory: the importance of human dignity* (Westport, Conn.: Praeger, 2002), R. Fjellstrom, 'Is Singer's ethics speciesist?', *Environ. Values,* 12/1 (2003), 91–106.

[19] Michael Tooley, 'Abortion and Infanticide', *Philosophy & Public Affairs,* 2/1 (1972), 37–65.

a right to life on the sole basis that they already exist as human beings. He argues that no one can have a right to something they are not aware of or have any desire to possess: '*A* has a right to X' is roughly synonymous with '*A* is the sort of thing that is a subject of experiences and other mental states, A is capable of desiring X, and if A does desire X, then others are under a prima facie obligation to refrain from that would deprive him of it'.[20]

When it comes to the right to life, Tooley suggests that the human infant is *not* 'A'. He believes that an infant lacks the equipment to be 'the subject of experiences and other mental states'; at least those that are relevant to desiring to live. Or, if she possesses the equipment, she has not yet learnt to use it. Either way, Tooley believes that the infant has no conception of herself as a living identity and so has no desire to possess life. There is, of course, a point in the development of normal human beings where the necessary equipment arrives and is usable, and it is at that point, Tooley suggests, that individuals acquire the right to life because they meaningfully prefer to be alive than dead. He suggests that this might be as early as a week of age. There is no sense, he argues, in which an infant under that age can be said to have a right to life, and parents should have the right to kill their infant during that first week of life if they so choose.

There is some variation in what theorists consider to be the exact nature of the infant's cognitive shortcomings. Tooley's defence of infanticide is on the grounds of his belief that, unlike an adult, the infant is as unaware of being deprived of life as those colour-blind tenants would be of the greyness of their walls. Peter Singer and Alberto Giubilini make similar claims, based, respectively, on their assessments of an infant's inability to formulate rational preferences and to have hopes for the future.[21] Underlying all three claims is the same presupposition that, in order for the moral agent to be as concerned about the interests of an infant as he would be about those of an adult, it would be necessary for the infant to appreciate the world and her own existence in the same way that an adult would. Such theories cannot accurately evaluate infants and children, because an adult-normative bias is 'hard-wired' into them. Any consequentialist theory that starts with the assumption that the ideal way for a human to exist is as an adult must inevitably privilege the properties and capacities that characterise the normal adult over those that characterise the normal infant.

---

[20] Ibid., p. 29. Tooley's proposition has been refuted in several different ways. John Stevens points out that a patient with a medical condition of which he has no conception might nevertheless have a right to be treated for it. Christina Sommers makes the deontological argument that, in becoming parents, adults take on a moral responsibility to care for a living child (C. H. Sommers, 'Tooley's immodest proposal: Abortion and Infanticide', *Hastings Cent Rep,* 15/3 (Jun 1985), 39–42.). Mark Tushnet and Louis Seidman suggest that, even if the infant herself has no right to live, killing her might transgress the rights of relevant others (M. Tushnet and L. M. Seidman, 'A comment on Tooley's Abortion and Infanticide', *Ethics,* 96/2 (Jan 1986), 350–5.). See also Davis, Nancy. 'Abortion and Infanticide (Book Review).' The Philosophical Review 94, no. 3 (1985): 436–441.

[21] Peter Singer, *Practical Ethics.* and Giubilini and Minerva, 'After-birth abortion: why should the baby live?'.

6.2.2 Removing the Safety Harness

A final reason for concluding that it is in the context of consequentialist moral theories that adult-normative thinking presents a particular danger to infants and children is that many traditional, non-consequentialist protections are removed. An exclusively consequentialist approach to bioethics does not just incur the risk of misclassifying infants and children as valueless; it also does away with some of the moral 'checks and balances' that medical ethics has traditionally offered. To a certain extent, the value of infants and children has historically been protected by some non-consequentialist moral theories. Even though deontological and virtue ethics accounts typically fail to ascribe inherent value to childness, they are less exposed to the risks that accrue from adult-normative bias because their account of personal value does not rely solely on capacities in the patient. The prejudicial effect of adult-normative thinking is attenuated, for example, in theories that frame ethical behaviour as a commitment to behave towards patients in ways that are disciplined by moral duties arising from professional obligations. The duties and obligations that result from such a commitment stand irrespective of whether or not a specific individual patient might be able to benefit from that behaviour.

Principlism, as we have seen, draws on several different theories. Its deontological claims in particular accommodate ideas of duty towards individuals who lack any capacity at all to benefit from correct moral decisions. The benefits that notions of honour and compassion offer to actual patients are often numinous and difficult to measure. Nevertheless, such ideas of correct behaviour represent ways of protecting infants and children by ensuring that they are treated in practice as though they had inherent value. Those protections are lost in a wholly consequentialist approach to medical ethics.

6.3 Summary

Traditionally, the value of infants and children was seen to be a function of the obligations, affections or capacities of adults. While such adult-normative accounts of personal value fail to accord inherent value to the infant or child herself, they have protected infants and children by appealing to non-consequentialist values such as the agent's own disposition and obligations. They are not a fix for adult-normativity, but they have offered a 'work-around' that enabled doctors to ascribe value to patients who lack the capacities of adultness as though they possessed inherent value.

Since the middle of the twentieth century, however, doctors have increasingly been schooled to base their practice on research evidence and to expect to be able to measure the effectiveness of an intervention by assessing its outcome. Rather than defining ethical behaviour in terms of obligations and duties that an honourable doctor will recognise, consequentialist moral theories frame it as a question of how much benefit such behaviour will offer in practice. According to consequentialism, the rightness or wrongness of a doctor's action is coextensive with the ability of the patient to benefit or to be harmed by it. That means the doctor's obligation to concern herself with the interests of a patient is determined by the patient's capacities. The extent of that obligation is determined by what desirable outcome is the objective of the consequentialist theory in question. A theory whose desirable object is to maximise satisfaction of rational preferences, for example, will privilege capacities necessary for reason and logic in the moral patient.

Most consequentialist theories are convincing when they offer an explanation as to why an individual possesses personal value. They are less reliable, however, when they conclude that an individual entirely lacks value. Most consequentialist theories are reductive; that is, they are aimed at maximising an outcome that is narrowly defined (such as happiness, or liberty, or preference satisfaction) so that the rightness of an action is expressible as a common denominator that can be calculated arithmetically by a process of adding benefits and subtracting harms. The soundness of a consequentialist moral theory aimed at improving the quality of human existence, however, depends on its capacity to recognise the full range of capacities that can permit an individual's existence to be meaningfully improved. It therefore depends too on the extent to which the theory correctly identifies an outcome that represents such a meaningful improvement. Consequentialist theories whose objective reflects too restricted a way of enjoying existence will easily misclassify individuals as non-persons or persons of no value.

Adult-normative thinking represents a specific way in which the desirable outcome can be too narrowly considered. Since the range of ways in which human existence can be improved is extremely wide and varied, it is difficult in practice to capture an outcome that is broad enough to be meaningful. Logically, the fact that the *presence* of certain capacities can confer value does not of itself require that their *absence* sets personal value at zero. In practice, however, many consequentialist bioethicists have concluded that the ideal way for humans to exist is as an adult, and that an individual human is of no inherent value if she lacks some or all the cognitive capacities that characterise the normal adult. A theory that connects moral value with certain personal capacities on the one hand, and on the other is committed to an adult-normative conception of what improves the quality of existence, inevitably under-values childness. It must also under-value an individual to the extent that he possesses childness.

How should the paediatric medical ethicist respond? We can first acknowledge, as Principlism does, that outcome is not all that is morally relevant; that there are also compelling explanations of value from deontology and virtue ethics. But we have already seen that even those explanations, while in practice offering children some protection, often reference adult-normative values and avoid the question of inherent value in childness itself. We have also seen that, notwithstanding the structural flaws of consequentialism, consequential thinking is a popular and valuable tool for analysing practical problems in medical ethics. Furthermore, where consequentialist accounts of personal value are unsatisfactory, it is because they are incomplete, rather than because they are incoherent. Where consequentialism *can* give an account of inherent value, that account is often compelling. We should not abandon consequential thinking.

When it comes to the value of infants and children, however, we should certainly be constructively sceptical about the objective of specific consequentialist theories. If a consequentialist theory is to evaluate an individual accurately, it must be sure it has correctly identified what capacities are morally relevant. The consequentialist theories that dominate medical ethics at the moment systematically undervalue infants and children, because they evaluate an individual's capacities by reference only to an adult's conception of what meaningful existence should be like. Consequential thinking can offer an explanation of childness' inherent value, but only if it sets aside that adult-normative bias and does not restrict its idea of the capacities that matter morally to those that permit someone to experience existence in the way that an adult does.

Whilst there is nothing in the structure of consequentialism itself that is inherently prejudicial to infants and children, the dominance of some specific consequentialist theories that currently influence medical ethical thinking presents some dangers in practice. One is that their effect is to express personal value entirely in terms of the capacities an individual possesses, and they are therefore confident in assigning a value of zero to anyone who lacks those capacities. A second is that they evaluate those capacities according to an adult-normative conception of what an individual needs to be able to do in order to exist meaningfully. A third is that they dismiss many of the ethical accounts that have traditionally protected infants and children, on the grounds that they appeal to non-consequentialist values.

In order to avoid those risks, a consequentialist theorist who wishes to justify evaluating an individual on the basis of her capacities must first get the outcome right; that is, she must select as an objective for medical ethics something that meaningfully represents human flourishing. She must also be sure that she is empirically correct about what she believes those capacities to be; clearly, if a moral agent's obligations to an individual depend on that individual's abilities, then it is important for the agent to assess those abilities accurately. Finally, while it is important for bioethicists of any philosophical persuasion to avoid systematic bias in their accounts of personal value, it is perhaps particularly important for consequentialist bioethicists since the latter express personal value only in terms of the nature of the patient, rather than in the duties or dispositions of the doctor. In the next three chapters, we will consider each of those in turn.

Paediatric bioethics should be sceptical about most of the best-known consequentialist moral theories, without dispensing altogether with consequentialism itself. We should acknowledge the power of consequentialism to ascribe value to certain cognitive characteristics, while at the same time interrogating carefully and critically its power to *deny* such value.

Bibliography

Agar N. How to insure against utilitarian overconfidence. Monash Bioeth Rev. 2014;32(3–4): 162–71.

Aristotle. Nicomachean ethics, Cambridge texts in the history of philosophy; trans. Crisp R. Cambridge: Cambridge University Press; 2000.

Bentham J. An introduction to the principles of morals and legislation. Principles of morals and legislation. Oxford: Clarendon Press; 1879.

Camosy C. Engaging with Peter Singer. In: Perry J, editor. God, the good, and utilitarianism: perspectives on Peter Singer. Cambridge: Cambridge University Press; 2014.

Fjellstrom R. Is singer's ethics speciesist? Environ Values. 2003;12(1):91–106.

Giubilini A, Minerva F. After-birth abortion: why should the baby live? J Med Ethics. 2013;39(5):261–3.

Harris J. Euthanasia and the value of life. In: Keown J, editor. Euthanasia examined: ethical, clinical and legal perspectives. Cambridge: Cambridge University Press; 1995.

Holm S. The peaceable pluralistic society and the question of persons. J Med Philos. 1988;13(4):379–86.

Koenigs M, et al. Damage to the prefrontal cortex increases utilitarian moral judgements. Nature. 2007;446(7138):908–11.

Krantz SF. Refuting Peter Singer's ethical theory: the importance of human dignity. Westport: Praeger; 2002.

Kuhse H. The sanctity-of-life doctrine in medicine: a critique. Oxford: Clarendon Press; 1987.

Long TA. Two philosophers in search of a contradiction: a response to Singer and Kuhse. J Med Ethics. 1990;16(2):95–6.

Mill JS. Utilitarianism. London: Longmans, Green and Co.; 1879.

Mill JS. A system of logic, ratiocinative and inductive: being a connected view of the principles of evidence and the methods of scientific investigation. Peoples ed. London: Longmans, Green, Reader, and Dyer; 1884.

Sidgwick H. The complete works and select correspondence of Henry Sidgwick (Sidgwick, complete works and select correspondence). Charlottesville: InteLex Corporation; 1996.

Singer P. Practical ethics. New York: Cambridge University Press; 2011.

Sloane A. Singer, preference utilitarianism and infanticide. Stud Christ Ethics. 1999;12(2):47–73.

Sommers CH. Tooley's immodest proposal: abortion and infanticide. Hast Cent Rep. 1985;15(3):39–42.

Tooley M. Abortion and infanticide. Philos Public Aff. 1972;2(1):37–65.

Tushnet M, Seidman LM. A comment on Tooley's abortion and infanticide. Ethics. 1986;96(2):350–5.

Williams BAO. A critique of utilitarianism. In: Smart JJC, Williams BAO, editors. Utilitarianism: for and against. Cambridge: Cambridge University Press; 1987.

Chapter 7
What Actually Matters

Humans have always been prone to separating people into categories with greater and lesser value. We tend to divide the world into 'in groups' of those whose interests we consider to be more important—usually people like ourselves—and 'out groups' of those whose value we consider to be less. Such divisions are rarely rooted in anything objective.[1]

We have seen that consequentialist moral theories in particular do not shrink from ascribing different values to different groups of humans. Their claim of most is that they are right in some objective sense to make such disparate evaluations, because they are made on the basis of something that is true, or at least agreed, about the groups in question. Following the publication of early editions of *Practical Ethics*, preference utilitarian Peter Singer professes himself astonished to find that many people drew parallels between his account of personal value and that of the Nazis.[2] He protests that, of course, he is in no doubt that the Nazis acted in a way

---

[1] Evidence suggests that some of the strongest factors influencing the emergence and definition of in- and out-groups lack any kind of objective significance in themselves: 'Cultural boundaries have often been the basis for discrimination, nationalism, religious wars, and genocide … arbitrary symbolic markers, though initially meaningless, evolve to play a key role in cultural group formation and ingroup favoritism because they enable a population of heterogeneous individuals to solve important coordination problems'.

[2] Singer, *Practical Ethics*, p. viii. See also Peter Singer, 'Bioethics and academic freedom', *Bioethics*, 4/1 (Jan 1990), 33–44. The protests were orchestrated, and largely carried out, by people with disabilities who felt his views legitimised and perpetuated societal judgements about the lack of value of their own lives. Singer dismissed those concerns because they: '… failed to point out that my views are no threat to anyone capable of expressing a preference for continued life, and thus obviously no threat to anyone capable of commenting on what I have written or said.' Later in the same article, Singer chooses to blame religious fundamentalism for his reception: 'Bioethics is a discipline that leads to the questioning of values and ethical doctrines that had previously been treated as sacrosanct. Often these doctrines are closely connected with religious beliefs, and we did not need Khomeini to remind us that religious fundamentalism is often intolerant of free speech' (Ibid., pp. 43–44).

R. Hain, *Childness and the Myth of the Unfinished Human*,
https://doi.org/10.1007/978-3-032-12111-0_7

that was morally indefensible.[3] But that is not, in his view, because Nazis considered it reasonable to kill some humans. Indeed, he manifestly embraces the same conclusion that humans who lack certain characteristics are not persons and can be killed at the behest of others.[4] The reason Nazis were wrong, Singer insists, is that the criteria they used to decide what sort of humans it was reasonable to kill were not the right criteria. Their conclusions were morally wrong because they were not adequately justified by rational argument or empirical demonstration.[5]

On consequentialist terms, an individual's value (considered as the extent to which a moral agent should concern herself with the interests of that individual) represents the extent to which the individual is equipped to suffer from the action in question. An invasive medical intervention that might be reasonable in a patient who could not experience pain, for example, might be morally impermissible if it were done to someone who could. In relation to medical ethics in children, a coherent consequentialist position would be that an adult-normative position is justifiable, *but only to the extent that adultness enables an individual to be harmed in ways that childness does not.*

The challenge for consequentialism is that the nature of harm itself cannot be defined without reference to the way in which humans ideally experience their existence. 'Harm' means broadly that well-being is jeopardised; but in order to recognise that jeopardy we have to have some sense of what well-being looks like in the first place. In order to consider the impact of childness on personal value on consequentialist terms, it is first necessary to consider how persons appreciate their own existence and which aspects of human cognition might therefore be relevant to being a person.

7.1 A Brief History of Personhood and What Might Matter to It

There is a sense in which a review of the ways in which philosophers and theologians have sought to distinguish 'person' from 'non-person' would, in effect, be a review of the whole of moral philosophy; perhaps even the entirety of philosophy itself and as such would be well outside the scope of this book. Fortunately, there are some themes on which philosophers' thinking has converged. The starting point for most utilitarian consequentialist accounts of personal value is John Locke's

---

[3] Singer, *Practical Ethics*, p. 21.
[4] Ibid., p. 167.
[5] Ibid., p. 155.

thoughtful definition of 'person'—as distinct from 'human being'—in *An Essay Concerning Human Understanding:*

> … to find wherein *personal Identity* consists, we must consider what *Person* stands for…. which, I think, is a thinking intelligent Being, that has reason and reflection, and can consider itself as itself, the same thinking thing in different times and places….[6]

Locke's main interest is in how persons think about themselves and each other. The point he is making here is that identity, and especially personal identity, consists in form rather than in material. There is an old joke about the gardener who comments that: 'I've had exactly the same spade for 20 years. In that time, it's had four new handles and three new blades'. The gardener is obviously correct in his belief that the spade remains the same spade. The fact that none of the original wood or metal remains is essentially incidental to its continuing identity as his spade, which consists in his own memory of it.[7] A person is a person, Locke says, because over time he continues to see himself as such.

One effect of Locke's definition is that it sets out the cognitive capabilities that a human being would need in order to possess personal identity on the terms he has laid out. They are the cognitive capabilities she needs to think, to be intelligent, to reason, to reflect, to know that she exists as an individual being and to remember what has happened in the past. That has led some to consider those capabilities to be a set of qualifications for the status of person. Philosopher Joseph Fletcher, for example, does not flinch from the conclusion that there are humans who fail to qualify, and he believes it is fairly easy to define who they are.[8] He distils 15 pass/fail criteria, of which he considers IQ (intelligence quotient—largely a measure of a faculty for logic) to be the most important.[9] That sort of thinking is broadly consequentialist, in that it takes for granted that a non-person will be harmed less than a person by being killed. But it does not establish a direct connection between the rightness of moral action on the agent's part and a capacity to suffer or be made happy. The assertion that only an individual who passes certain tests qualifies as a

---

[6] Locke, *An Essay Concerning Human Understanding Book II: Ideas*, p. 115. He goes on to add the idea that a person is accountable for making morally correct choices: 'Person, as I take it, is the name for this self. Wherever a man finds what he calls himself, there, I think, another may say is the same person. It is a forensic term, appropriating actions and their merit; and so belongs only to intelligent agents, capable of a law, and happiness, and misery' (Ibid., p. 120).

[7] Trigger reaches the same conclusion about his road-sweeping broom in an episode of 'Only Fools and Horses' and Plutarch gives a more highbrow illustration of the same idea using Theseus' ship, whose sails and planks are replaced one by one over many years but which most people (including, we assume, Theseus himself) would have continued to see as Thesus' ship.

[8] Joseph F. Fletcher, *Humanhood: Essays in Biomedical Ethics* (Prometheus Books, 1979), pp. 12–16.

[9] 'Any individual of the species *Homo sapiens* who falls below an IQ grade of 40 in a standard Stanford-Binet test, amplified if you like by other tests, is questionably a person; below the mark of 20, not a person. *Homo* is indeed *sapiens* in order to be *Homo*' (Ibid., p. 12). On the basis of IQ alone, Fletcher would consider as 'questionable' persons around a third of those with Down's Syndrome and around one human in a hundred who has no pathology but is simply at one end of the IQ distribution among the population of normal humans.

person needs clearly to explain why, on those grounds, a moral agent's obligations to a person are different from her obligations to a non-person. What is it about someone who has an IQ less than 40 that diminishes a moral agent's obligations to her? What is it about being *sapiens* that imposes obligations on the moral agent that would not be imposed otherwise?

Peter Singer supplies one answer in *Practical Ethics*. Singer applauds Fletcher's general approach to defining moral status and, without granting the implication that they are the sole preserve of members of the species *Homo sapiens*, he agrees that Fletcher's list successfully captures the attributes that are morally important.[10] He sets out a form of utilitarianism that expresses all the cognitive abilities he considers important to personal value in one criterion: the capacity to hold a preference. A meaningful preference, he points out, demands sophisticated thought processes such as understanding, reflection and deliberation.[11] The distinction that Fletcher makes between person and non-person is represented in Singer by the difference between individuals capable of holding such preferences and those capable only of having interests. Interests, he suggests, arise out of a broader and less choate expression of subjective experience than preferences do.[12] To have interests, it is only necessary to possess the capacity to suffer.[13] The cognitive abilities necessary to qualify an individual for personhood, on that view, are those that enable an individual to develop preferences; that is, hypotheses about what will enable her to be happier or to avoid suffering. A being who is incapable of holding preferences might be able to suffer but, according to Singer, he is a non-person.[14]

Despite his approval of Fletcher's account of personhood and his own focus on preference satisfaction as the desirable outcome of moral action, Singer reserves his wholehearted endorsement for the idea of personal or biographical narrative.[15] Philosopher Gary Varner suggests that what makes human persons distinctive is that we continually construct explanations for what our senses tell us about the world and our relationship with it.[16] This desire to create narrative about ourselves on the one hand, and possession of the cognitive equipment and capacities to be able to do so on the other, permit what Varner calls a 'biographical sense of self'. The term refers to meaning-making; the way that each of us connects together what we see, hear and feel about the world in order to make some kind of sense of it, and of our place in it. Varner suggests that ultimately it is the impulse and ability to construct a

---

[10] Singer, *Practical Ethics*, p. 176.

[11] Ibid., p. 14.

[12] 'Intelligence has nothing to do with many important interests that humans have, like the interest in avoiding pain, in satisfying basic needs for food and shelter, to love and care for any children one may have, to enjoy friendly and loving relations with others and to be free to pursue one's projects without unnecessary interference from others' (Ibid., p. 22).

[13] Ibid., p. 50.

[14] Ibid., p. 48.

[15] Ibid., p. 122.

[16] Gary E. Varner, *Personhood, ethics, and animal cognition: situating animals in Hare's two level utilitarianism* (New York; Oxford: Oxford University Press, 2012), p. 134.

biographical sense of self that represents the only categorical difference between human reasoning and the reasoning of non-human animals. The impulse to construct such an explanation arises primarily from our need to organise our sensations, which does not depend on the explanations mapping precisely onto what is actually true, so that the story we tell ourselves need not be accurate in any objective sense.

Some philosophers have sought to link personhood to an ability to speak, on the grounds that moral reasoning represents a form of dialogue with oneself.[17] Varner suggests that although speech is relevant to biographical narrative, it need not be dependent on it: '[Reasons for considering humans to be special] have little to do with the standard candidates for a uniquely human ability: rationality, tool use (or tool making), and language. I think that what makes humans special has something to do with language, but it is not having language per se. Rather … it is telling stories about our lives and our cultures'. Varner is suggesting that what distinguishes person from non-person is *not* that persons possess the capacity for reasoning or language, but that reasoning and language are important when they result in the construction of narrative meaning.[18] The concept of biographical life does not rule out the possibility that there are other ways of constructing such a narrative that do not rely on a capacity for speech.

Personhood, on that account, is a complex form of appreciative existence. It represents a constructivist engagement with the world by means of subjective sensations, and an individual is a person if she possesses the capacities that allow her to construct explanations for what she senses about herself and about the world.[19] The idea of biographical life as an indicator of personal value has gained wide acceptance in bioethics. It is appealing to many consequentialists because it offers a plausible link between the rightness of an agent's action on the one hand and, on the other, the various capacities the subject of that action might possess that would allow her to benefit from or be harmed by it. Biographical narrative is also attractive to those who are troubled by consequentialism's vulnerability to overly restricted definitions of the desirable outcome of moral action, because it substantially avoids the risk of an excessively reductive approach to saying what exactly those capacities are. Properly considered, the concept of narrative or biographical life is as capacious as the concept of flourishing. Like flourishing, the idea of biographical life can ascribe value to almost any of the ways in which an individual appreciates and engages with the rest of the world.

---

[17] See, for example, D. C. Dennett, *Brainstorms: philosophical essays on mind and psychology* (Penguin science; London: Penguin, 1997), p. 285.

[18] Varner, *Personhood, ethics, and animal cognition: situating animals in Hare's two level utilitarianism*, p. 134. Peter Singer wrongly suggests that Varner considers a capacity for biographical life to be reliant on an ability to speak. Singer, *Practical Ethics*, p. 103.

[19] Philosophy and medicine have given different meanings to the word 'perceive'. In medicine, perception is a physiological term which refers to a reflexive response by nerve cells that does not engage any higher cortical centres. In philosophy, on the other hand, 'perception' is often taken to mean something that represents an individual's reflective interpretation of their sensations. The difference between reflexive and reflective are so important in this context that I have chosen to avoid the term 'perception' wherever possible.

In contrast to the readiness of other consequentialist theories to set personal value at zero, there is little risk that a theory whose objective is to improve the quality of an individual's biographical narrative will mis-classify someone as a 'non-person'. The concept of personhood that biographical narrative represents is so capacious and complex that it defies precise delineation. The number and variety of ways in which an individual might construct a meaningful biography is enormously wide, and it would be impossible to compile a comprehensive list of the cognitive skills and abilities that might allow her to do so.

It would be especially hard to identify with confidence someone who was entirely *unable* to do it. The only clear 'fail' criterion, perhaps, would be an individual who lacks the physical equipment necessary for cognition of any kind. The first prerequisite for a biographical narrative is that an individual must possess the necessary organs. Constructing a biographical life is like driving a car: you cannot do it, or even learn how to do it, if you do not have the necessary equipment to start with. Here we have an advantage over Aristotle, whose conclusions about when humans acquired a rational soul were limited by the fact that he was relying on anatomical dissections and did not know which organ was necessary for reasoning. We have now identified that organ.[20] It is the brain, we now know, that is responsible for the logic, feelings and emotions that connect what an individual senses to the way she explains or experiences it.

There are cognitive skills and capacities whose presence indicates an ability to construct a meaningful biographical narrative. The most obvious is an impulse or desire to do so. Owning a car is not the same as actually driving it; before being considered a driver, you need to want to get into the car and set off. Understanding that there is something that demands an explanation in the first place, and possessing an impulse to construct a narrative that explains it, are what constitute biographical life. Thereafter, biographical narrative is, broadly speaking, a matter of being aware of oneself, being aware of the world outside oneself (and especially other people in it) and having the habit of constructing hypotheses to account for connections between them.

---

[20] For the purposes of this discussion I am assuming that there is a duality between mind and body, which maps precisely onto a distinction between brain and non-brain organs. There is intriguing evidence that that is only broadly true, and that some aspects of what we consider 'mind' might be housed in other organs. Paul Pearsall, Gary E. R. Schwartz, and Linda G. S. Russek, 'Changes in heart transplant recipients that parallel the personalities of their donors', *Integrative medicine: integrating conventional and alternative medicine,* 2/2 (2000), 65–72. See also J. A. Armour, 'The little brain on the heart', *Cleveland Clinic journal of medicine,* 74/Suppl_1 (2007), S48.

7.1.1   *Being Aware of Oneself*

There is a conception that an infant is entirely unaware of herself as an individual, which seems to have its roots in a Victorian view articulated by physiologist William James who wrote in 1890 that: '[A]ny number of impressions, from any number of sensory sources, falling simultaneously on a mind which has not yet experienced them separately, will fuse into a single undivided object for that mind. … The baby, assailed by eyes, ears, nose, skin, and entrails at once, feels it all as one great booming, buzzing confusion'.[21] The nature of self-awareness, insofar as it is relevant to biographical narrative, is contentious. A capacity for biographical narrative is implied by an individual's awareness of herself, both as *distinct from* other persons and *in relation to* them. Singer draws a helpful distinction between sentience and self-awareness. A sentient being can suffer or experience pleasure, but only a being who is self-aware can hold a preference to continue to live.[22] Exactly what being 'self-aware' means, however, is unclear. Peter Singer appears to believe that an individual demonstrates everything that is morally relevant about self-awareness if he passes the mirror self-recognition test.[23] The mirror test was the work of biopsychologist Gordon Gallup, who developed it in the late 1960s to assess self-awareness in non-human animals.[24] It consists in making a mark on some part of an animal's body that the animal can only see in a mirror. The animal is then given access to a mirror, and is said to possess self-awareness if it demonstrates that it realises the mark is on its own body. Gallup's research was important because it revealed a clear distinction between great apes, most of whom who 'pass' the test, and monkeys, who all 'fail' it.

It is far from clear that the test demonstrates anything meaningful in humans. There are many different ways in which distinctness from others might be conceived, from a capacity for complete isolation from the influence of others on the one hand to the mere recognition that others occupy a different physical space from oneself on the other. Summarising the conclusions of a series of his own studies into self-awareness, cognitive neuropsychologist Valéry Legrain comments that a person is aware of herself in a number of different ways simultaneously: 'Our results

---

[21] William James, *The principles of psychology* (Authorized edn., Dover books on philosophy and psychology; New York: Dover, 1950). It is interesting that in those early pre-psychology days James considers the infant's obliviousness to result from a state of over-alertness and excessive receptiveness rather than representing the infant in the way that Tooley, Singer and Giubilini did eight decades later as *lacking* in important forms of awareness.

[22] Singer, *Practical Ethics*, p. 65.

[23] 'Self-awareness … has been tested by putting a coloured dye on a part of the animal where it will be seen in the mirror but cannot be seen otherwise–for example, on an ape, the forehead. (The dye is put on when the animal is asleep so that she does not notice.) Then the animal is given a mirror, with which she has previously become familiar. If she looks in the mirror and then touches the dyed spot, this indicates that she knows that the image in the mirror is herself'. Singer, *Practical Ethics*, p. 101. Singer's summary here is accurate.

[24] G. G. Gallup, Jr., 'Chimpanzees: self-recognition', *Science,* 167/3914 (Jan 2 1970), 86–7.

support the notion that self-awareness is not a monolithic, all-or-none ability'.[25] We can understand that by imagining a man walking down a rainy street in London. He will be aware of the physical boundaries of his own body, and what happens when the wind and rain of the material universe interact with those boundaries. He will be aware of his physical sensations of coldness and wetness, and he will be aware that they concern him in a way that the coldness and wetness of others do not. He might also commence an internal dialogue along the lines of how unlucky he is, imagine how much better his life would have been if there had been no tube strike, and anticipate with pleasure the warm bath he will have when he gets home. Those reflections are all forms of self-awareness. But they are quite different from one another, and demand quite different cognitive capacities from the individual.

Philippe Rochat, an experimental psychologist at Emory University in the United States, explains that there are many ways of passing the mirror test, some of which have little to do with self-awareness per se: '… there are different ways of passing the test, including solipsistic, nonsocial ways'.[26] Rochat goes on to say that 'Interestingly, multiple studies demonstrate that neurodivergent subjects who pass the mirror mark test do so with flat affect, displaying "completely neutral" expressions, with no signs of either coyness or embarrassment,' which might suggest that self-recognition represents no more than a logical acknowledgement of one's existence. On the basis of what is known about which sides of the brain are associated with different intramental functions, Canadian experimental psychologist Alain Morin concludes that what 'passing' the mirror test demonstrates is the kinaesthetic aspect of self-awareness, rather than consciousness of one's existential self through self-description ('How wet and cold I am') or through autobiography ('How much better my life would have been if the tube trains were running, and how much better it will be when I get home and have a hot bath').

The heterogeneous nature of self-awareness is important. There is clearly a morally important distinction to be made between self-descriptive and autobiographical self-awareness and the mere awareness of one's physical position or movements in space. 'Organisms that display MSR [mirror self-recognition]' says Morin, 'most probably do not possess introspective self-awareness'.[27] That idea of 'introspective self-awareness' seems to be close to Locke's characterisation of a person as

---

[25] L. Legrain, A. Cleeremans, and A. Destrebecqz, 'Distinguishing three levels in explicit self-awareness', *Conscious Cogn,* 20/3 (Sep 2011) pp. 578–79.

[26] Philippe Rochat, Tanya Broesch, and Katherine Jayne, 'Social awareness and early self-recognition', *Conscious Cogn,* 21/3 (Sep 2012), 1491–7 p. 1496.

[27] A. Morin, 'Self-recognition, theory-of-mind, and self-awareness: what side are you on?', *Laterality,* 16/3 (May 2011), 367–83. That piece of evidence alone casts serious doubt on Singer's claims about personhood in infants and some of his assumptions about nonhuman persons. Morin's view is supported by the observation that Capuchin monkeys who are not self-aware can be trained to pass the mirror test (see P. G. Roma et al., 'Mark tests for mirror self-recognition in capuchin monkeys (Cebus apella) trained to touch marks', *Am J Primatol,* 69/9 (Sep 2007), 989–1000). Presumably the Capuchin monkeys are learning the movements needed to pass the test, rather than acquiring existential self-awareness.

possessing '… reason and reflection, [who] can consider itself as itself'.[28] If personal value relies on that sort of self-awareness, then, according to Morin and Rochat, it seems difficult to argue that the mirror test demonstrates anything relevant to it at all.

Moreover, even if it were still agreed that passing the mirror test probably demonstrates the *presence* of relevant awareness, it would be fallacious to conclude on that basis alone that failing the test reliably demonstrates the *absence* of such awareness.

7.1.2 Being Aware of Others: Relationality

The life of any individual person is inextricably bound up with the lives of others, and the ability to acknowledge and process those relationships is evidence of a capacity for biographical narrative.[29]

One way to look at relationality is to express it merely as the cognitive skills an individual needs in order to be able to engage with other individuals. That would put a capacity for relationality on all fours with, say, a capacity for logical reasoning. But, considered as a capacity relevant to personal value, relationality is different from other capacities in one important respect: it inherently requires awareness of at least one other person. The faculty of logic is self-contained. It can be exercised without any reference to another individual, and even without acknowledging the existence of such another individual. The capacity for logic is analogous to the sound a car's engine makes. Every car with an engine makes its own noise; there is no need for any other car to exist in order for that noise to happen. By analogy, there is no need to reference the existence of any other person in order to conclude that a particular person has a capacity for logic. Relationality, on the other hand, expresses not only the capacity to *have* relationships, but an acknowledgement that such relationships are possible because other people exist. Relationality entails plurality.

The understanding that other people exist, moreover, represents a relationship in itself. The capacity for relationality is like the sound of cars crashing into one another. The question 'which car made the sound of the crash?' is nonsensical, because the sound only happened because they collided. The sound exists because two or more cars have come into contact and, without that interaction between them, there would be no sound at all. A capacity for relationality represents more than an individual's possession of the necessary cognitive equipment. It represents the fact that she is already in such relationships and knows herself to exist in the context of them.

---

[28] Locke, *An Essay Concerning Human Understanding Book II: Ideas*, p. 115. Ibid., p. 120.

[29] Even Peter Singer includes 'the capacity to relate to others' among the criteria for personhood. Singer, *Practical Ethics*, pp. 181–82. That does not obviously cohere with his preference utilitarian claims elsewhere that only a capacity to formulate preferences, based on rationality and self-awareness, can confer personal value.

A *capacity for* relationality expresses an individual's acknowledgement of others and, as such, it represents an interaction and is already *evidence of* relationality. That is important because, on those terms, relationality does not merely express possession of the equipment and capabilities necessary to form relationships. Nor does it express the idea that a person's value is reliant on the value given to them by others by virtue of a specific relationship or sort of relationship (such as a loving relationship between mother and child). Relationality is awareness of the reality that every individual person exists in interaction with other persons.

7.1.3   Being Able to Create Connections Between Cause and Effect

Constructing a biographical narrative is a way of discovering order. It describes establishing some connection between various experiences and sensations of the world. That can be a process of inductive reasoning, concluding that such-and-such is the reason for so-and-so, or merely the observation that, in practice, when such-and-such happens, the result is always so-and-so. Discovering order requires a capacity to regulate the flow of incoming data. Construction of an effective narrative sometimes demands a 'horizon-scanning' approach to sensation, which opens up the filter to include as much new data as possible, while at other times it demands narrowing of the filter so that extraneous data is excluded and the individual can focus on specific parts of it.

The kind of constructivism that biographical life represents is a form of learning. An awareness of one's own past and future implies an ability to construct a biographical narrative, permitting a process of reviewing hypotheses that have been shaped by previous sensations and amending them in the light of current ones, and is permitted by an ability to retain data about sensations long after the sensations themselves have ceased—in other words, memory. A capacity for registering and recalling what sensations tell us, both about the world in general (incidental memory) and about specific elements within it (endogenous memory), is evidence of an ability to construct biographical narrative.

7.2   Summary

It is not only card-carrying consequentialists who realise that, when it comes to behaving ethically, outcome matters. Nor do we have to agree that an agent's obligation to others extends only as far as others' capacity to benefit or suffer in order to accept that cognition is morally relevant. We do not have to capitulate to the idea that patients with an IQ less than 40 lack value or are 'non-persons' in order to agree that there are circumstances under which someone's cognitive abilities are relevant to how we should treat them.

A colleague once told me of a particularly challenging post-graduate exam for which I was preparing that no one passed who should fail, but plenty of people failed who should pass. The same might be said of the various criteria for person-hood that have been proposed. Seen as a 'pass' mark when they are present, they are usually plausible; it is obvious that the presence of certain cognitive capacities imposes an obligation on the moral agent to concern herself with an individual's interests. No one doubts, for example, that a patient who possesses the capacities needed to make an autonomous decision should be offered the chance to do so. Consequentialist thinking poses a risk, however, if the absence of such criteria is seen to be a 'fail' mark. Under those circumstances, pass/fail criteria carry the risk of wrongly setting someone's personal value at zero, suggesting that the moral agent need not concern herself with an individual's interests at all. I have suggested in an earlier chapter that the risk posed to children is particularly high because the adult instinct is to recognise the value of adultness more easily than that of child-ness. An effective defence against such mis-evaluation, of course, is to acknowledge non-consequential sources for personal value, such as compassion or dignity. Without abandoning the consequentialist commitment to evaluating individuals on the basis of their capacities, the only way to mitigate the risk of mis-valuing is to be certain that we have accurately assessed those capacities and their moral relevance.

If we are to take on the task of evaluating individuals on the basis of certain cog-nitive capacities, the capacity to construct a biographical narrative offers a particu-larly plausible yardstick for assessing them. The desire to narrate appears to be a distinctively human one, and biographical narrative represents something that is both agreed by a broad 'church' of moral philosophers and is sufficiently capacious to avoid the dangers of an over-reductive account of what enables humans to flourish.

I have set out several capacities whose presence indicates that an individual is able to construct such a biographical narrative. The requisite anatomical equipment, and the impulse to use it, are necessary, though not sufficient. Awareness of self, awareness of others and a habit of constructing narrative on the basis of such aware-ness are all indicators of personal value on consequentialist terms because they are ways in which the individual's experience of her life is made meaningful. In the next chapter, we will consider ways in which the cognitive capacities we now know childness to encompass can permit the construction of such a biographical narrative.

The list is permissive, not exhaustive. The capacious conception of what consti-tutes a meaningful existence that biographical narrative represents means that, even on consequentialist terms, the range of capacities that is relevant to personal value is much broader than Locke has allowed. There are, for example, adult patients whose memory extends back only a few minutes and, while their ability to construct narrative is different from that of others or their former selves, they continue to engage with the world and to make meaning of what they sense. There are many cognitive faculties that can undoubtedly help someone flourish when they are pres-ent, but that does not entitle us, even on consequentialist grounds, to relegate some-one else to the status of non-person simply because they are absent.

Bibliography

Armour JA. The little brain on the heart. Cleve Clin J Med. 2007;74(Suppl_1):S48.

Dennett DC. Brainstorms: philosophical essays on mind and psychology, Penguin science. London: Penguin; 1997.

Efferson C, Lalive R, Fehr E. The coevolution of cultural groups and ingroup favoritism. Science. 2008;321(5897):1844–9.

Fletcher JF. Humanhood: essays in biomedical ethics. Prometheus Books; 1979.

Gallup GG Jr. Chimpanzees: self-recognition. Science. 1970;167(3914):86–7.

James W. The principles of psychology, Dover books on philosophy and psychology. Authorized ed. New York: Dover; 1950.

Legrain L, Cleeremans A, Destrebecqz A. Distinguishing three levels in explicit self-awareness. Conscious Cogn. 2011;20(3):578.

Locke J. An essay concerning human understanding book II: ideas. Jonathan Bennett; 2004.

Morin A. Self-recognition, theory-of-mind, and self-awareness: what side are you on? Laterality. 2011;16(3):367–83.

Pearsall P, Schwartz GER, Russek LGS. Changes in heart transplant recipients that parallel the personalities of their donors. Integr Med. 2000;2(2):65–72.

Rochat P, Broesch T, Jayne K. Social awareness and early self-recognition. Conscious Cogn. 2012;21(3):1491–7.

Roma PG, et al. Mark tests for mirror self-recognition in capuchin monkeys (Cebus apella) trained to touch marks. Am J Primatol. 2007;69(9):989–1000.

Singer P. Bioethics and academic freedom. Bioethics. 1990;4(1):33–44.

Singer P. Practical ethics. New York: Cambridge University Press; 2011.

Varner, G.E. (2012), Personhood, ethics, and animal cognition: situating animals in Hare's two level utilitarianism (New York/Oxford: Oxford University Press).

Chapter 8
Solvitur Ambulando: Turning to the Evidence

In this chapter on empirical evidence, I will focus largely on the infant, by which I mean a child in the first year—more often in the first few days or weeks—of life. Earlier I suggested that most children are cognitive 'hybrids' who, as they make their way from birth to adulthood, owe their way of appreciating and engaging with the world at any one time both to childness and to adultness, in proportions that change as the child grows older and in response to her life circumstances. The newborn infant is an exception to that general rule, because he has yet to acquire any of the cognitive characteristics of adultness. It is thus the infant whose cognition illustrates childness in its most nearly pure form. In searching for what empirical science tells us about the nature of 'childness', it is to research in infants that we primarily need to turn. That should not, of course, be taken to mean that such research tells us nothing about the older child, because the older child too demonstrates childness, though not usually to the same degree as the infant.

8.1   The Danger of Projection

In his argument for what he calls 'after-birth abortion', Alberto Giubilini asserts that '… the future we imagine for [a newborn] is merely a projection of our minds on its potential lives'.[1] There seems little doubt that Giubiini is right that, in their interactions with babies, the usual reaction of adults is to try to interpret what is going on

---

[1] 'If … an individual is capable of making any aims (like actual human and non-human persons), she is harmed if she is prevented from accomplishing her aims by being killed. Now, hardly can a new-born be said to have aims, as the future we imagine for it is merely a projection of our minds on its potential lives. It might start having expectations and develop a minimum level of self-awareness at a very early stage, but not in the first days or few weeks after birth'. Giubilini and Minerva, 'After-birth abortion: why should the baby live?'.

R. Hain, *Childness and the Myth of the Unfinished Human*,
https://doi.org/10.1007/978-3-032-12111-0_8

inside the baby's head. Certainly, anyone who has been a friend of new parents will attest to the prone-ness of proud parents to overestimate the capacities of their infant. We are quick to see a deliberate smile in a quiver of our own baby's lips that could equally easily be wind, or to tell ourselves she is choosing to hold our finger when in fact it is a reflex grasp.

The converse, of course, is also true. There are circumstances under which adults are prone to *underestimating* an infant's actual capabilities. For many years, for example, adults believed firmly that infants lack the equipment to feel pain. It was a belief that probably originated in a 1941 study, in which neonates were repeatedly pricked with a pin while the investigator noted the way in which the babies' responses changed over time.[2] On the basis of her observations, the study's author Myrtle McGraw concluded that the infant has no more sensation of pain than that of an anaesthetised adult.

Over the course of the decades that followed McGraw's study, it became clear that her conclusions were quite wrong. We know now that newborn infants unquestionably do feel pain, in substantially the same multimodal way that adults do.[3] McGraw had wrongly interpreted what she saw. She knew already that the system of pain perception in infants was slightly different from adults, and assumed that the difference would mean it did not work as well as that of an adult. She assumed too that pain in a normal infant would look the same to an observer as pain in a normal adult. It was a sophisticated form of projection: McGraw made her observations through an adult-normative lens, with the result that they endorsed and even reinforced beliefs about the infant that she already held. Later studies that set aside those presuppositions were to show that the differences between adult and infant nerves mean the infant experiences more pain, not less.[4]

It is easy for philosophers, as well as scientists, to project their own presuppositions onto the object of their study. Since she cannot correct us, there is little to prevent us from drawing conclusions about an infant's cognition that are more confident than is strictly justified by the evidence. The risk of underestimating what an infant understands and can experience is perhaps greater than the risk of exaggerating it, because something we know for certain about the infant is that, to a great extent, she lacks control of her body. The way infants in McGraw's study responded physically to a pin-prick was, as she observed, similar to the way in which an adult would respond if he were deeply anaesthetised. But that was not because the infants were less capable than adults of experiencing pain; it was because they were less able to control the movements they made in response to it. The infant's obvious

---

[2] M.B. McGraw, 'Neural maturation as exemplified in the changing reactions of the infant to pin prick', *Child Development,* 12/1 (1941), 31–42. One assumes the study ended at the point where the children became big enough to hit back.

[3] S. Goksan et al., 'fMRI reveals neural activity overlap between adult and infant pain', *Elife,* 4 (2015).

[4] Anand and Carr, 'The neuroanatomy neurophysiology and neurochemistry of pain stress and analgesia in newborns and children', *Ped Clin N Am,* 36/4 (1989), 797–822, Anand and Hickey, 'Pain and its effects on the human neonate and fetus', *NEJM,* 317/21 (1987), 1321–29.

motor incompetence offers a parallel temptation to adults to assume she is equally incompetent when it comes to cognition. Infants cannot speak, so they cannot tell us what they are feeling or experiencing. That is not simply because they lack the muscular control to form words physically, but because they have not yet learned to clothe concepts in words in the first place.[5] Speech is the only way that most individual humans can communicate with any precision what they are feeling and, until recently, there was no other way of accessing an individual's subjective experience. Without being able to interrogate verbally what an infant is experiencing, it is difficult for adults to avoid projecting their own prior beliefs onto what they observe. If you already believe the infant to be merely sentient in theory, that is the way in which you will interpret what you observe about the infant in practice. The infant cannot tell you one way or another whether or not you are correct.

The point can be illustrated by imagining that, say, an entirely rational and self-aware philosopher awakes one morning to find that overnight he has had a stroke. Unusually, but perfectly plausibly, he finds he has retained his ability to see and hear. His ability to reason too remains intact, but his only movements are involuntary; he cannot control them and as a result can no longer talk. When his colleagues break into his house to see why he has not appeared in the lecture hall, it would be quite natural for them to assume that, since he can no longer demonstrate that he is experiencing life, or possesses a mental state, or desires to live, the philosopher no longer experiences life, possesses a mental state, or desires to live. And it would be difficult to disprove their assumption empirically. Nevertheless, their assumption would not be objectively correct. Nor (more importantly for the purposes of this discussion) would it be a rationally valid conclusion for them to draw from what they observe once they know that the professor is unable to move, because that inability already fully explains what they see. It would be fallacious for the professor's colleagues to infer from their observation of his motor deficiencies that their unfortunate friend is also unable to experience, or to possess a mental state, or to desire to live, because experience, possession of a mental state, or a desire to live are not contingent on motor ability, nor are they plausibly connected to it. A motor deficit that prevents an individual from communicating the fruits of cognition must not be taken as evidence of a deficit in cognition itself. Aphasia does not in any way imply dementia.

Infants are at considerable risk from adult projection of narratives of incompetence. The idea that newborn infants cannot feel pain became accepted wisdom and, for much of the twentieth century, babies were routinely operated on while

---

[5] There is an important distinction between the capacity for speech, which is merely making words, and a capacity for language. In his analysis of Piaget's work, moral philosopher Charles Taylor links a child's language capacity with her capacity to make meaning (Charles Taylor, *The language animal: the full shape of the human linguistic capacity* (Cambridge, MA: The Belknap Press of Harvard University Press, 2016), p. 4.). Taylor concludes that language is not just an instrument for expressing or marshalling ideas that a child already has, but rather, that the acquisition of language permits the child to make 'new purposes, new levels of behaviour, [and] new meanings' that would otherwise be impossible. That making of meaning constitutes a form of reasoning.

conscious and without pain relief.[6] That was agreed by most adults in society to be a morally correct way of responding to infants because it was—or appeared to be—a rational and compassionate approach. Anaesthesia during surgery carries definite risks, especially in the first weeks of life. If infants cannot experience pain, that risk would be hard to justify and it would be wrong to administer anaesthetics. But as a matter of fact they can feel pain. Withholding anaesthesia was an act of appalling cruelty, to which people who were compassionate and rational were drawn because they had misinterpreted what they observed, and were consequently misinformed in ways that mattered to the moral decisions they made.

Giubilini's assumption is that infants lack the cognitive capacities necessary to value their own life in the present moment, and he is clearly convinced that any other belief an adult might hold about the infant is illusory. McGraw probably felt the same about any instinctive reluctance surgeons had about operating on infants without anaesthesia in the last century. But without an appeal to empirical evidence, it is equally possible that it is Giubilini, and those who think like him, who are projecting.

8.2 The Availability of Evidence

Writing in the latter part of the twentieth century, Peter Singer is another adherent to Tooley's account of infant cognition. Singer lists what he considers to be the capacities that are necessary in order to be harmed, and which he believes are encompassed by adultness, but not childness: 'The embryo, the later fetus, the profoundly intellectually disabled child, even the new-born infant … none are self-aware, have a sense of the future, or the capacity to relate to others'.[7] Elsewhere, he reiterates his belief that the infant lacks self-awareness: 'Neither the fetus nor the new-born infant is an individual capable of regarding itself as a distinct entity with

---

[6] It has been astonishingly tenacious. In 1987, one correspondent to the New York Times wrote: 'Your article on infant pain and its belated recognition by the medical community (Science Times, Nov. 24) suggests that unanesthetised surgery has been limited to newborns and that the practice had largely ended by the late 1970's. However, surveys of medical professionals indicate that as recently as 1986 infants as old as 15 months were receiving no anesthesia during surgery at most American hospitals' (Helen Harrison, 'Why Infant Surgery Without Anesthesia Went Unchallenged', *New York Times*, 17th December 1987, p. A34). As recently as 2011, developmental psychologist Philippe Rochat commented that: 'Even today, local anesthetics are not routine in painful procedures on newborns such as heel prick and circumcision, even by pediatricians practicing in state of the art maternity hospitals. The Zeitgeist continues to be that infants have either no feelings, less feelings, or that feeling experience at this early stage might not be as consequential for lack of memory (infantile amnesia)' (Philippe Rochat, 'The self as phenotype', *Conscious Cogn,* 20/1 (Mar 2011), 109–19 p. 111). The idea that it is acceptable to allow someone to experience pain providing they do not remember it is clearly problematic, though perhaps it coheres with some conceptions of personal value as continuous identity.

[7] Singer, *Practical Ethics*, pp. 181–82.

a life of its own to lead…'[8] On that basis, Singer believes that infants, like objects, '… have no interests to be considered'.[9]

Singer's authority is Roman philosopher Seneca, whose: '… compassionate moral sense strikes the modern reader (or me, anyway) as superior to that of the early and mediaeval Christian writers, [and who] also thought infanticide the natural and humane solution to the problem posed by sick and deformed babies'.[10] Seneca's evaluation of infants was understandable when Seneca held and expressed it in the first century. Like Aristotle before him, he was writing at a time when no one really knew what children thought or felt before they were able to talk. That lack of research data continued to dog moral philosophy in respect of infants well into the twentieth century and when, in 1972, Tooley first promulgated his theory that that infants less than week old are not equipped to experience their lives in any way that amounts to a desire to continue living, no one knew whether, as a matter of fact, it was correct. Theories regarding the cognitive processes of childness were difficult to prove or to refute scientifically, and perhaps at the time it did not seem even hypothetically possible that we would ever know what went on in the minds of humans who cannot speak or control their own muscles. The citations in *Abortion and Infanticide* are all references to philosophical works rather than to research articles in journals of developmental psychology, neurology or paediatrics. They represent beliefs, not knowledge. Tooley acknowledges that, as the science of human neuro-development progresses and more empirical evidence becomes available, his argument in respect of infanticide will stand or fall by the objective truth about infant cognition that such research uncovers. He seems to have been in no doubt that such evidence would corroborate his account. His confidence is so great, in fact, that he even suggests that science will indicate that an infant's state of non-personhood continues for longer than the week that he has proposed.[11]

Time was to prove Tooley at least partly correct. He was right to anticipate that in the following years important new evidence would appear which would inform the argument he had made for infanticide. Over the last 20 or 30 years, techniques have been developed that now render it possible to make objective observations about the workings of the infant mind.[12] Tooley's confidence that new evidence

---

[8] Ibid., pp. 164–65.

[9] Ibid., p. 106.

[10] Ibid., p. 153.

[11] '[Because] it is virtually certain that an infant at such a stage of its development does not possess the concept of a continuing self, and thus does not possess a serious right to life, there is excellent reason to believe that infanticide is morally permissible in most cases where it is otherwise desirable. … the practical moral problem can thus be satisfactorily handled by choosing some period of time, such as a week after birth, as the interval during which infanticide will be permitted … This interval could then be modified once psychologists have established the point at which a human organism comes to believe that it is a continuing subject of experiences and other mental states'. "Tooley, 'Abortion and Infanticide'.

[12] The advent of functional magnetic resonance imaging in the early 1990s was particularly important, allowing researchers to identify which parts of the brain are functioning during certain actions or thoughts. It is, in effect, becoming possible to 'read the mind' of some individuals who are

would support the beliefs that he held in 1972 was, however, misplaced. Far from confirming the view that Tooley held, by the time Singer sought to disinter Seneca's understanding of infants and bring its influence to bear on bioethics in the 1980s, research was already revealing that infants are cognitively much more capable than had hitherto been assumed. The more we have learnt about the infant, the more we have realised he is cognitively capable of doing. In the period that has elapsed since *Abortion and Infanticide* appeared, there has been a substantial body of relevant research in respect of self-awareness in the human infant. The weight of evidence that has accumulated overwhelmingly militates against Tooley's 1972 assertion.[13]

The question is perhaps not yet entirely beyond doubt. Modern techniques, sophisticated though they are, do not yet allow us to access the specific thoughts of pre-verbal infants. They do, however, provide some evidence in respect of the similarities and differences between infant and adult thinking that does not always depend, as it has in the past, on inferences on the part of investigators. Alison Gopnik is a neuropsychologist and philosopher whose doctoral research in Oxford in the late 1970s examined the development of the concepts behind language, including self-awareness and awareness of what is 'non-self', in children between 1 and 2 years old. Over the past three decades, Gopnik has carried out a series of studies in developmental psychology. In her book, entitled *The Philosophical Baby: What Children's Minds Tell Us About Truth, Love and the Meaning of Life*, Gopnik reviews the results of her own empirical research and that of others in the field in order to set out what the intervening decades have taught adults about the way an infant perceives the world, and how she sees herself in relation to it.[14] As the title suggests, Gopnik's main conclusion is that the normal infant's cognition, while quite distinct from the cognition of adults, is a highly effective tool for human meaning-making.

One of Gopnik's central observations about childness concerns a difference in the ways adults and infants are aware of the world. Research evidence shows that, while an adult's awareness is typically focused on the detail of what he perceives, an infant's awareness is aimed at eliciting as much data as possible about the universe, as quickly as possible and from as many sources as possible. Gopnik dubs these different forms of awareness 'spotlight' consciousness and 'lantern consciousness'. Spotlight consciousness illuminates intensely the specific things on which it focuses but leaves other things completely dark. 'Lantern' consciousness

---

physically unable to articulate words. There are several examples. fMRI has, for example, allowed individuals to spell out words without movement (Bettina Sorger et al., 'A Real-Time fMRI-Based Spelling Device Immediately Enabling Robust Motor-Independent Communication', *Current Biology*, 22/14 (7/24/ 2012), 1333–38). There are ways of enabling those who have lost the power of speech to control voice-synthesisers using their brain alone, though at present they still require the patient to have previously had the capacity to form words physically (H. Akbari et al., 'Towards reconstructing intelligible speech from the human auditory cortex', *Sci Rep*, 9/1 (Jan 29 2019), 874).

[13] Goksan et al., 'fMRI reveals neural activity overlap between adult and infant pain'.

[14] Alison Gopnik, *The Philosophical Baby: what children's minds tell us about truth love & the meaning of life* (London: Bodley Head, 2009).

illuminates everything equally, though the light that falls on any one area is relatively dim. Spotlight consciousness is schooled by (and therefore, to a certain extent, limited to) what a person already expects to see and considers to be important, while lantern consciousness makes no such prior assumptions. Gopnik considers that the greater reach of lantern awareness permits the infant to perceive more of the universe than the adult:

> Babies are more conscious than we are. They are ceaselessly and broadly engaged in the kind of information-processing and learning that adults direct only at limited, relevant events. And babies are less subject to the processes that actively cause unconsciousness in adults–inhibition and habituation.[15]

Although 'lantern' awareness characterises childness and is most obvious in infants, adults can know what it is like because we too sometimes experience it in our own appreciation of the world. It is lantern awareness, for example, that informs us about the world in a new country during the taxi ride from the airport to the hotel on the first day.[16] Things that are mundane and would normally go unnoticed force themselves on our attention, whether or not we are looking for them, because we have not seen them before. Unfamiliar makes of car are driving on the wrong side of the road, signposts are in different colours and are written in a foreign language, the buildings look odd and there are species of tree and flower that are entirely new to us. It soon passes but, while it persists, adults are experiencing something of what an infant experiences all the time.

Much more often, according to research, adults demonstrate spotlight consciousness, which allows us to focus on a small part of what is around us and to perceive it in great detail. There are, of course, circumstances under which that is clearly preferable. As an airline passenger, what I want the pilot to bring is a precise and logical understanding of the plane's controls and the physics of flight, and a reluctance to be distracted from the task of flying the aeroplane. The awareness that characterises adultness is nevertheless, in a sense, much more limited than what characterises childness, because it focuses on a subset of data in order to consider it carefully and so restricts the scope of what is perceived.

All that makes developmental sense. An individual person needs to be able to garner information about the world in one way when she is a newcomer to it, and in a different way when she has had some experience of it. At first, the main existential priority is to gather as much information as possible as quickly as possible, and an individual's need is to cast the net of her awareness as widely as her organs of sensation will allow. A lantern-style way of appreciating the world achieves that. Later on, as the individual begins to construct theories and narratives to explain how it all connects and what it all means, it becomes more important to direct those sense

---

[15] Alison Gopnik, 'Why babies are more conscious than we are', *Behavioral and Brain Sciences,* 30/5–6 (2007), 503–04 p. 504.

[16] 'When adults are placed in a situation that is functionally similar to babies, such as traveling in a strange country or meditating in certain ways, we experience a similarly vivid but distributed phenomenology–consciousness becomes a lantern instead of a spotlight'. Gopnik, *The Philosophical Baby.*

organs to solicit specific data that can support and expand such theories and narratives.

8.2.1 Children and Narrative: Capacities in Common

By the time the infant reaches 10 or 11 months of age, we are aware that he is beginning to tell his own story. He is already able to play the part of an adult; he will recognise that a doll represents (but is not actually) a baby, and that in such a representation the infant himself stands in respect of the doll as a parent does to a baby, that the way a parent should relate to a baby is to hug them, and that all this is not 'real' in the same sense that the infant himself is real. They are extraordinarily complicated constructions of meaning about the universe in which the infant exists that depend on a capacity to learn, to identify with (and care for) other humans, and to form and value relationships. The older infant is clearly 'one of us', engaged as we are in constructing a biographical narrative.

What about the younger or newborn infant? She certainly possesses the necessary equipment. The newborn brain is smaller than the adult brain, but otherwise anatomically little different. The cortex, which is the part of the brain specialised for cognition, is a little thinner, the folds or sulci of the brain's surface somewhat shallower, and a greater proportion of an infant's nerve cells have yet to acquire the myelin sheath, which speeds up nerve transmission. On the other hand, the nerve cells in an infant brain possess a capacity for synaptogenesis—literally, making connections—and plasticity (generating new nerve cells where needed in response to what is sensed) that the adult brain has largely lost. Given the constructivist nature of biographical narrative, that capacity for making connections suggests the infant is at least as well equipped for biographical narrative as the adult is. Of course, possessing the equipment needed to construct a narrative is not enough on its own to show that the infant is actually engaged in doing so. There is also evidence that young infant humans, like adults, are drawn to telling their own story. Psychoanalyst and clinical psychologist Peter Fonagy uses the term 'subjective self' to represent the idea of biographical narrative in infants and reviews the evidence that the desire to develop it is strongly developed from birth.[17]

Whether or not the human infant possesses self-awareness is more contentious. Peter Singer suggests that the infant's ability to experience the world is the same as

---

[17] 'A central characteristic of these models of primary "intersubjectivity" is a shared emphasis on the continuity from infancy to adulthood of subjective emotional experience, of the kinds of "intersubjective" states of interpersonal relatedness, and of the identity of basic human motives that are supposed to drive the mutual affect-regulation and attunement assumed to characterise dyadic interactions from the beginning of life'. P. Fonagy, G. Gergely, and M. Target, 'The parent-infant dyad and the construction of the subjective self', *J Child Psychol Psychiatry*, 48/3–4 (Mar–Apr 2007), 288–328 p. 292.

that of a late fetus.[18] It appears from *Practical Ethics*, however, that he believes the human fetus experiences nothing at all.[19] It is not always easy to obtain a clear or consistent understanding of the moral status which, on those terms, Singer feels we should accord to humans during infancy. If the fetus has no relevant consciousness at all, then it must have no interests and is in the same category as a stone. And if Singer is right that the cognitive processes of the fetus and the newborn baby are the same, then it seems he should infer that the infant too can have no experiences and so has no more interests than a stone. On that basis, he would have to conclude that it would be ethically acceptable for a boy to kick a baby down the street, providing her parents did not object; certainly, on that view, it would be more acceptable to kick a baby than to kick a mouse. There is nothing in Singer's writing to suggest that he believes any such thing, but it is not clear why, since in order to avoid such a conclusion he would have to concede either that the fetus and the baby are both conscious, or else that the cognitive abilities of the infant are relevantly different from those of the fetus, both of which he seems to deny.[20]

Singer's difficulty in remaining consistent with an account of personal value that equates the awareness of fetuses and newborn infants with that of stones is partly the result of what he understands self-awareness to represent. Singer understands self-awareness to be something of which the infant is as manifestly bereft as a billiard ball is of hair.[21] The powerful, if uncomfortably facetious, imagery he chooses to use leaves no doubt that Singer understands self-awareness to be a capacity that the infant utterly lacks. He seems persuaded that all rational people agree with him, and with his Tooleyean claim that the condition persists until some weeks or months after birth. His confidence in such universal agreement flows from his conviction that it has been empirically proven by means of the mirror test. He compares the performance of the human infant in the test unfavourably with that of some animals,

---

[18] 'Now we have to face the fact that these arguments apply to the new-born baby as much as to the fetus'. Singer, *Practical Ethics*, p. 151.

[19] 'The fetus itself, if killed before awareness commences, experiences nothing different than it would have experienced if it had not been conceived–for in both cases there are no experiences at all' (Ibid., p. 142).

[20] Singer's position here can be made consistent by recognising that there is a point in each individual fetus' development at which awareness develops. On utilitarian terms that is the point at which the fetus becomes sentient for the first time. Since Singer believes (albeit wrongly) that the individual then remains sentient, but not self-aware, until the end of infancy, he can argue consistently that the moral value of infants and [late term] fetuses are the same. Elsewhere, he concedes that the infant (and therefore, presumably, the late term fetus) is capable of experiencing pleasure and suffering and on that basis accords her the inherent value of a 'merely conscious' being (Ibid., p. 85).

[21] 'It would, of course, be difficult to say at what age children begin to see themselves as distinct entities existing over time. But a difficulty in drawing the line is not a reason for drawing it in a place that is obviously wrong, any more than the notorious difficulty in saying how much hair a man has to have lost before we can call him "bald" is a reason for saying that someone whose pate is as smooth as a billiard ball is not bald ....' (Ibid., p. 153).

noting particularly the remarkable abilities of an African grey parrot named Alex.[22] Singer believes that failing the mirror test demonstrates conclusively that self-awareness is absent and, since the capacities of childness do not enable the normal human infant to pass the mirror test, he assumes that they do not enable the infant to be self-aware in any way that would allow the infant to construct a biographical narrative.

Singer's main target in bioethics is the casual anthropocentric assumption that all humans, and only humans, should be the object of moral concern. He is therefore keen to separate the idea of personal value from the idea of species. The mirror test suits that polemical purpose, because it not only measures something that is plausibly related to personhood; it also turns out to be something that some non-humans can do, while some humans cannot: 'All the great apes can pass the mirror test … Human children less than one year old typically fail the mirror test, but by the time they are eighteen months old, most can pass it'.[23] Singer takes this to be empirical proof that infant humans lack self-awareness, and when the first edition of his *Practical Ethics* was published in 1979, that was a reasonable interpretation of what was known.[24]

Barely 5 years later, further research had demonstrated that human infants of 2 or 3 months old are self-aware even if they had 'failed' the mirror test.[25] There are particular potential confounding factors in interpreting the mirror test in humans.

---

[22] 'All the great apes can pass the mirror test … Pepperberg's meticulously recorded account of [Alex's] abilities and behaviour leaves little doubt that he too was self-aware to some extent. Human children less than one year old typically fail the mirror test, but by the time they are eighteen months old, most can pass it' (Ibid., p. 102). This seems to be the only empirical evidence Singer adduces in his argument that human infants are not self-aware. The scale of some of the changes in moral behaviour that utilitarians are willing to advise on the basis of abstract theorising causes New Zealand philosopher Nicholas Agar some concern: 'I accuse those who seek to translate these conclusions into moral advice of a dangerous overconfidence'. Agar, 'How to insure against utilitarian overconfidence', p. 162.

[23] Singer, *Practical Ethics*, p. 102. Singer's reluctance to subject his beliefs about the infant to more rigorous empirical scrutiny suggests a readiness to abandon reason for polemic. The general willingness of utilitarian philosophers to recommend significant changes in practical moral behaviour on the basis of abstract lines of reasoning alone causes New Zealand philosopher Nicholas Agar some concern: 'I accuse those who seek to translate these conclusions into moral advice of a dangerous overconfidence'. Agar, 'How to insure against utilitarian overconfidence', p. 162.

[24] A painstaking review of empirical evidence around self-recognition, carried out by psychologist James Anderson only a few years after *Practical Ethics* was published, suggests that it was then generally accepted by authorities in the field that passing the mirror test indicates a form of awareness that humans do not demonstrate until after they have left infancy: '… there is general agreement surrounding certain aspects of the infant's developing ability to recognize itself. For example, mirror-guided responding to otherwise invisible marks, which must be based on self-recognition, does not occur before 15 months of age, emerges in some infants shortly thereafter, and is characteristic of most infants by the age of 2 years'. J. R. Anderson, 'The development of self-recognition: a review', *Dev Psychobiol,* 17/1 (Jan 1984), 35–49 p. 47. It is noteworthy that as early as 1984, Anderson chooses not to comment on the relationship between self-recognition, self-awareness and personhood.

[25] Anderson, 'The development of self-recognition: a review'.

Some of the reasons for failing the test result from characteristics such as sociality that are relevant to moral agency and are well-developed in the human infant. For example, children are less likely to respond to the spot on their forehead if the investigator himself has a spot too.[26] By the time the 2011 edition of *Practical Ethics* appeared, it had been clear for some decades that Singer's confidence in the mirror test was misplaced. He recognises that for an animal to fail the test does not reliably exclude self-awareness but in 2011 does not acknowledge the same limitation when it comes to the test's inability to exclude self-awareness in human infants.[27]

Among developmental neuropsychologists, James' nineteenth-century conception of childness as a state of 'one great booming, buzzing confusion' has long ago been consigned by science to obsolescence.[28] On the day she is born, an infant already knows herself to be physically distinct from the rest of the universe.[29] She knows herself too to be distinct from other individuals. She has already developed the concept of 'contingency'; she understands that, even though they look the same, there is an important difference between a being whose body she can control and one that she cannot. On the first day of life, infants already distinguish their own touch from that of others.[30] The infant's sense of awareness of self goes beyond a sense of physical separation from others. Infants less than a day old respond

---

[26] '[When parent and researcher were marked in addition to the child], children displayed significantly more hesitation while removing the mark, often touching it without removing it or, if so, promptly putting the mark back onto their forehead. In the Classic condition, only one child showed such hesitation. These results suggest that from the outset, mirror self-recognition can refer to social awareness. This link is interpreted as the trademark of human self-consciousness, a deeply rooted "looking glass" self- awareness'. Rochat, Broesch, and Jayne, 'Social awareness and early self-recognition'.

[27] 'Passing the mirror test may show self-awareness but failing it does not prove that an animal is not self-aware'. Singer, *Practical Ethics*, p. 244.

[28] 'Recent empirical findings suggest that infants do not come to the world with the exclusive expression of self-obliviousness … Contrary to the assumption of many classic theories of child development, infants are not born in a state of fusion or confusion with environment (the "booming, buzzing, confusion" proposed by William James [in]1890)'. Philippe Rochat, 'Five levels of self-awareness as they unfold early in life', *Consciousness and Cognition*, 12/4 (2003), 717–31 p. 722.

[29] 'More recent research shows that, in fact, healthy newborns do perceive the world objectively and are not in a state of subject–object confusion. From birth they express a difference between what pertains to their own body and what pertains to the world "out there". Within the proposed framework, infants at birth do not just sense and respond based on reflex-like mechanisms'. More recent research shows that, in fact, healthy newborns do perceive the world objectively and are not in a state of subject–object confusion. From birth they express a difference between what pertains to their own body and what pertains to the world 'out there'. Within the proposed framework, infants at birth do not just sense and respond based on reflex-like mechanisms. Rochat, 'The self as phenotype', p. 114, Rochat, 'Five levels of self-awareness as they unfold early in life', p. 723.

[30] 'In a recent study, we compared [rooting] responses in 24 h old infants following either a tactile stimulation originating from the index finger of the experimenter or from self-stimulation, infants spontaneously bringing one of their hands in contact with a cheek. Systematic comparison shows that neonates do root significantly more to external compared to self-stimulation'. Rochat, 'Five levels of self-awareness as they unfold early in life', p. 722.

differently to recordings of their own voice from those of other babies of the same age.[31] That suggests a meaningful sense in which infants are self-aware that has nothing to do with visually recognising their likeness in a mirror. Passing the mirror test is not, in other words, the only way to demonstrate the sort of self-awareness that is relevant to biographical narrative.

Showing that a non-human animal can pass the mirror test is important because it provides convincing evidence of some sort of self-awareness. That makes it highly plausible the animal has the capacity to suffer, which, on the terms we are setting out, should concern a moral agent. The mirror test therefore certainly supports the idea that humans should treat non-humans better than we do. But it does not show that a human infant is not meaningfully self-aware, because an infant who is self-aware in ways that are relevant to constructing biographical narrative might nevertheless fail the mirror test. Whether awareness of self is considered merely as the exclusive occupation of a certain physical space, or as a more sophisticated existential distinctiveness from other individuals in the universe, empirical research makes it clear that it is within the compass of even the newborn infant.

We have seen that relationality is evidence of a capacity to construct biographical narrative; perhaps, in its own way, more important even than rationality. Relationality is a form of narrative construction in itself, which depends on a certain sort of awareness of oneself and of others as well as an understanding of the interplay between them. Research has shown that an individual's awareness that he exists in relation to others is part of the way the human brain becomes 'hard wired' during foetal development.[32] By the time he is born, a human's understanding of the universe already includes a 'person network' that embraces the infant himself and other humans.[33] Research also shows that the sort of narrative of interdependence, of which infants are highly capable, can be the basis for constructing a meaningful biography.[34] The suggestion that the newborn infant lacks such a capacity would in any case be improbable on the face of it; it seems unlikely on evolutionary grounds

---

[31] Grace B. Martin and Russell D. Clark, 'Distress crying in neonates: Species and peer specificity', *Developmental Psychology,* 18/1 (1982), 3–9.

[32] 'The operation of an intrinsic motive formation (IMF) that developed in the core of the brain before birth is evident in the tightly integrated intermodal sensory-motor coordination of a newborn infant's orienting to stimuli and preferential learning of human signals, by the temporal coherence and intrinsic rhythms of infant behaviour, especially in communication, and neonates' extraordinary capacities for reactive and evocative imitation'. C. Trevarthen and K. J. Aitken, 'Infant intersubjectivity: research, theory, and clinical applications', *J Child Psychol Psychiatry,* 42/1 (Jan 2001), 3–48.

[33] '… a certain region of cortex is destined for face recognition as early as age 1 day, and other regions, which are capable of recognizing inanimate objects, cannot take over this function. This striking absence of plasticity implies that the category of human face, as well as its representation by specific brain tissue, is determined essentially at birth'. M. J. Farah and A. S. Heberlein, 'Personhood and neuroscience: naturalizing or nihilating?', *Am J Bioeth,* 7/1 (Jan 2007), 37–48 p. 43.

[34] Fonagy, Gergely, and Target, 'The parent-infant dyad and the construction of the subjective self', p. 288.

that infant humans could survive without being able to establish a relationship with humans who are older, stronger and more experienced. And if infants cannot survive, then neither can humankind. An infant constructs her biographical narrative on the basis of such a person network, of which she already sees herself and her parents to be a part.

8.2.2   Children and Narrative: Contentious Capacities

Of the six characteristics set out in the last chapter whose presence indicates a capacity to construct meaningful biographical narrative, we have now seen that four are shared even by the very young infant. At or immediately after birth, humans already possess the necessary anatomical equipment and are drawn to using it. They are aware of themselves in ways that are relevant to meaningful biography, albeit ways that are different from older children and adults, and they are aware of others in a way that not only demonstrates a capacity for relationality but in itself already constitutes a relationship.

Two remaining candidate capacities for personal value are more contentious: reason and awareness of time passing. We also need to consider the relevance of autonomy. A capacity for autonomy did not appear on the last chapter's list of capacities that permit biography, because its contribution to constructing narrative is represented by more basic capacities such as reason, self-awareness and—paradoxically perhaps—relationality. But, in medical practice, we have come to accord evaluative power to the capacities necessary for autonomy, to such an extent that some bioethicists consider those capacities to be coextensive with personal value.

These three facilitators of biographical narration—reason, futurity and autonomy—are particularly important in the context of medical ethics in children because they are capacities that mark adultness but do not obviously mark childness.

8.2.2.1   Reason

A challenge with considering reason as a contributor to personal value is that its meaning is far from agreed. It has been defined as the 'human ability to discover an underlying order in any field of inquiry'.[35] In the twenty-first century, it is often taken to be synonymous with a capacity for calculative and analytical logic which

---

[35] Theologian Anthony Celano, summarising what twelfth century theologian Thomas Aquinas understands by reason (Anthony Celano, 'Medieval Theories of Practical Reason: The Thomistic Doctrine of Practical Reason', *Stanford Encyclopedia of Philosophy*, https://plato.stanford.edu/entries/practical-reason-med/, accessed 1st March 2017.)

excludes, and may even stand in opposition to, emotions, intuitions and instincts.[36] In science, a theory is rational if each step is explained in some logically valid way by the one before, and medicine understands the term in that scientific sense. The World Health Organization (WHO), for example, defines 'rational' medical practice exclusively in terms of the need for careful logic in prescribing medications.[37] Providing the initial empirical observations are accurate, a theory is correct if the explanation it offers for those observations is logically consistent.

Such calculative logic, however, is not the only mode in which humans tell their own story. Considered as a contributor to biographical narrative, reason can be a much more capacious term that encompasses feelings and intuitions. Moral philosopher Susan Krantz points out reason can be understood '… broadly in two ways: (1) it may be understood as a calculative faculty, a logical activity, which determines what follows from what; or (2) it may be understood as a faculty of insight, an intuitive or insightful activity, which discerns the essence or nature of a thing'.[38] In relation to biographical life, one sense that 'reason' and 'rational' convey is the idea of getting the story right; constructing elements of personal narrative that are congruent with what is actually true, or at least with what seems to be true given what we have sensed or been told. We awake with heartburn and a headache and reach the conclusion that it is the result of having drunk too much the night before. We see an eclipse of the sun and attribute it to the anger of the gods in a way that makes perfect sense given our understanding of the universe at the time. The explanations may or may not be true in an objective sense, but they are logically consistent and as such can be considered rational.

While logical consistency is often helpful in discovering underlying order, it is not necessary in order for a narrative to be important to personal identity and value. Logic is not the only mode in which humans habitually find themselves reasoning, and if a capacity for reason were conflated entirely with a faculty for logic, then it would be easy to dismiss much of normal human cognition at any age as morally irrelevant. In practice, when it comes to constructing narrative, most individuals are likely to be influenced at least as much by how they feel as they are by what they can infer or deduce.[39] A 25-year-old man who experiences chest pain will usually

---

[36] Moral philosopher Barry Hoffmaster explains: 'The formal reason of philosophy is rule-governed reasoning, the kind of inferential reasoning used in logic and mathematics. This view percolates through ordinary understandings of rationality as well, exemplified by the familiar use of the expression, "That's not logical," to mean, "That's not rational." Deducing theorems from axioms in logic or geometry is a paradigmatically rational activity, and this paradigm can easily be extended to other domains so that the application of moral principles or rules of law to the facts of cases likewise is a paradigmatically rational enterprise'. Barry Hoffmaster, 'The Rationality and Morality of Dying Children', *The Hastings Center Report,* 41/6 (2011), 30–42 p. 30.

[37] '… patients [should] receive medications appropriate to their clinical needs, in doses that meet their own individual requirements, for an adequate period of time, and at the lowest cost to them and their community'. World Health Organisation, *Promoting Rational Use of Medicines: Core Components – W.H.O. Policy Perspectives on Medicines.*

[38] Krantz, *Refuting Peter Singer's ethical theory,* p. 35.

[39] See, for example, Hoffmaster, 'The Rationality and Morality of Dying Children', p. 30. 'Formal reason is not adequate to explain how we think through real-life problems and make moral decisions about them'.

assume correctly that the cause is indigestion or a bruised rib. But if he has recently lost his father to a heart attack, the narrative he constructs around the chest pain will be very different. That difference in biographical narrative is real, even though it cannot be explained on the basis of logic alone. It is hard to explain logically why people should choose to gaze at a painting, listen to music or—less comprehensibly still—decide to gather to watch 22 other people kicking a football around a field. It is hard to explain on the basis of logic what it is that attracts one person to another. But the fact that these behaviours are not logical does not alter the contribution they nevertheless make to the narrative that an individual constructs about his or her existence. Most observers would hesitate to claim that falling in love was not an important part of their biographical narrative.

While those are not rational behaviours, in the sense that they result from formal and logical reasoning, they could, perhaps, be described as reasonable. A distinction between what is reasonable and what is rational is intuitively clear, though it is difficult to explain etymologically, because it results from a conceptual gap between two ideas that are not distinguished in the Latin word ratio from which 'reason' and 'rational' both derive. Ratio can refer to reckoning in the sense of logical induction or deduction. But ratio can also refer to understanding, in the aesthetic sense of the way in which a being engages with the universe, including itself. Reasoning of that second sort would encompass a being's many modes of information-gathering through his senses, and the myriad forms of awareness that shape those perceptions into a narrative that makes some order of what he perceives.

We have already seen evidence from neurodevelopmental psychology that the infant is aware of relationships and is engaged in the development of the 'subjective self'.[40] The advent of functional magnetic resonance imaging (fMRI), which enables researchers to observe the brain's activity, has now made it clear that despite their immature nerve development, infants are capable of sophisticated reasoning of that intuitive and aesthetic sort. At 2 months, what the infant sees is already associated with activity in multiple, connected parts of the brain, indicating that he is making meaning on the basis of what his senses tell him.[41] When it comes to pain, such connections appear even earlier. An infant is trying to make sense of pain, in much the same way that an adult does, within the first 7 days of life.[42]

---

[40] 'It is suggested that the infant focuses on the attachment figure as a source of reliable information about the world. The construction of the sense of a subjective self is then an aspect of acquiring knowledge about the world through the caregiver's pedagogical communicative displays which in this context focuses on the child's thoughts and feelings'. Fonagy, Gergely, and Target, 'The parent-infant dyad and the construction of the subjective self', p. 288.

[41] Nathalie Tzourio-Mazoyer et al., 'Neural Correlates of Woman Face Processing by 2-Month-Old Infants', *NeuroImage,* 15/2 (2002), 454–61.

[42] Goksan et al., 'fMRI reveals neural activity overlap between adult and infant pain'.

8.2.2.2 Futurity and the Awareness of Time

Awareness of time passing, too, is ambiguous in ways that are relevant to the question of the contribution it can make to biographical narrative. There seems little doubt that memory can be important, since biographical narrative can represent a form of continuous identity that connects the present with the past. Some authors, however, have argued that in order for a meaning-making being to have full value as a person, that sense of continuous identity must also extend into a future that exists only in the imagination of the biographer.

So far, fMRI has not examined temporal perception in children younger than 8 years. There is, however, evidence that infants of only a month old already have a sense of time passing, and even a rudimentary sense of futurity.[43] We also know that the infant is well-equipped with memory. The infant possesses a sense of time passing, an excellent memory and an ability to learn, which argues for a sense of continuous identity in the Lockean sense which Singer endorses. Gopnik shows that, compared with older children and adults, the infant is particularly good at remembering information about the world in general.[44] One blow to the classical tabula rasa theory is evidence that babies have already laid down some memories by the time they are born. For example, at birth, babies have already acquired musical preferences and some aspects of their parents' accent, arguing that there is a very basic sense in which they have already started to construct some form of biographical narrative.[45]

It is less clear, however, that any infant possesses a capacity for what has been described as 'futurity'; that is, an individual's capacity to project herself into a situation that has not yet occurred. The awareness that futurity represents is something that occurs in the present moment, just as the memory of events past represents an awareness (and, on strictly materialist grounds, ultimately a conformation of physical molecules in the brain) that is occurring in the here and now. Futurity differs from memory, however, in that it is not linked to actual existence. A memory may

---

[43] Sylvie Droit-Volet, 'Time perception in children: A neurodevelopmental approach', *Neuropsychologia*, 51/2 (2013/01/01/ 2013), 220–34.

[44] '… infants develop endogenous attention much later, and it is still developing during the pre-school years. Moreover, and probably correlated with this fact, infants and young children appear to have less focused attention than older children–for example, they show better incidental memory'. Gopnik, 'Why babies are more conscious than we are'.

[45] 'There is compelling evidence that infants are sensitive to prosodic features of their native language long before speech-like babbling sounds are uttered or first words are produced. Indeed, auditory learning starts as early as the third trimester of gestation, and prosodic features are well preserved across the abdominal barrier, whereas phonetic aspects of speech are disrupted, making prosodic characteristics very salient for the human fetus. In newborns, traces of early auditory learning processes are reflected in perceptual preferences for melodies to which they were exposed prenatally … The observed melody contours of French and German newborns' crying show that they not only have memorized the main intonation patterns of their respective surrounding language but are also able to reproduce these patterns in their own production' (Birgit Mampe et al., 'Newborns' Cry Melody Is Shaped by Their Native Language', *Current Biology*, 19 (2009), 1994–97).

be incomplete or inaccurate, but it is usually a matter of objective fact that some version of a remembered event took place. A person's memory usually attaches to a moment that has actually happened, and in which that person actually existed. Futurity, on the other hand, relies entirely on speculation and reasoning based on prior experiences. The individual assumes she will exist into the future because she was alive in the past, and experience tells her that existence is continuous. A capacity for futurity requires both an understanding that the future exists, and that the individual herself exists in a way that will extend into that future. In that sense, futurity demands more complex cognition than remembrance of the past.

Some utilitarian philosophers hold that a sense of futurity is an indispensable attribute for constructing a biographical narrative.[46] In the same way that Locke considered personhood to represent a sense of continuity with one's past self, and therefore to be reliant on memory, some utilitarians argue that, when it comes to personal value, that sense of continuity must also extend into an individual's future and to rely on a capacity to appreciate that future. Importantly, the point here is not about an actual future, but about the idea of a future that an individual might have in the here and now. An individual is entitled to have that idea and, if he has it, then even on utilitarian terms it would usually be morally wrong to take it from him by killing him. The utilitarian argument is not seeking to make personal value reliant on shamanic powers of prevision, in other words, but on a present capacity.[47]

For those who wish to espouse infanticide, a defence of adult-normativity on the grounds of futurity is attractive because it links the concerns of the moral agent exclusively to a capacity that childness, as far as we know, does not encompass. The utilitarian consequentialist defence of infanticide represents an assertion that the capacities of childness do not allow their possessor to be harmed by being killed. If an infant cannot form a preference for continued life, then in deciding whether the infant should live or die, the agent need only consider the preferences of others.[48]

---

[46] For example, Singer, *Practical Ethics*, p. 122.

[47] A similar idea emerges in James Rachels' term 'realisable goals'. The goals themselves relate to events in the future, but the utilitarian value they confer on an individual's current existence is in the fact that they are held in the present moment (James Rachels, *The end of life: euthanasia and morality* (Studies in bioethics; Oxford: Oxford University Press, 1986), pp. 64–65).

[48] Though she can be harmed in other ways. A logical consequence of this line of reasoning is that the moral agent should concern herself with preserving an infant from experiencing pain, but need not concern herself with preserving the infant's life. Peter Singer is particularly anxious to make this distinction. Medical ethicist Andrew Sloane summarises Singer's position as follows: 'he claims [that] human infants, while clearly sentient, in that they can experience pleasure and pain, are not persons, for they are not rational, are unable to communicate, and have no sense of themselves as existing over time. Thus, while it is wrong, on preference utilitarian grounds, to cause an infant to suffer, it is not wrong to kill an infant. Indeed, in light of the preferences of the infant's parents not to rear, say, a disabled child, it may be permissible, even right, to kill the infant' (Sloane, 'Singer, preference utilitarianism and infanticide', p. 57). Sloane's summary is concise and correct, but in introducing the concept of personhood and the criteria of rationality, ability to communicate and a sense of self over time, Sloane slightly over-simplifies Singer's position and risks obscuring an important weakness in Singer's argument; namely his lack of knowledge about the cognitive processes of the infant.

Given the increasing sophistication of research techniques, it is perhaps not inconceivable that in the future we will be able to access humans' internal mental experiences, during infancy and outside it. At the moment, however, our capacity to do so is limited and, in contrast with arguments that invoke self-awareness, we cannot turn to empirical proofs to help refute arguments that invoke futurity and must rely instead on reasoning.

Singer seems to invoke biographical narrative to defend his belief that a sense of futurity is an indispensable attribute of personhood. The principal benefit of being alive in the present moment, he suggests, is the knowledge that one will continue to live into the future: 'Continued existence cannot be in the interests of a being who *never* has had the concept of a continuing self–that is, never has been able to conceive of itself as existing over time. If [a] train … instantly killed [an] infant, the death would not have been contrary to the interests of the infant, because the infant would never have had the concept of existing over time'.[49] That would locate the inherent value of a life entirely in its possessor's expectation that it should continue, which is problematic because it gives no value at all to the experience of being alive in the present moment. To pursue Tooley's analogy of car-ownership, locating the value of an individual's life exclusively in her preference that life should continue is like suggesting that the only joy I get from owning a car is the idea that I will still own it tomorrow. That disregards any pleasure I might already be having by driving it today. It is surely nonsense to suggest that my pleasure in owning the car is expressed wholly in my reluctance for it to be taken from me at some later date. It is equally bizarre to suggest that the only reason for not taking my life today is that, all other things being equal, I expect and prefer to continue to have it tomorrow.

Varner, originator of the idea of biographical narrative, agrees. He explains that an individual's life story today is shaped, not only by her hopes about what might take place in some notional future, but also by her lived experiences in the past and present.[50] Today, at this moment, I am rejoicing in being alive and everything that being alive allows me to experience. A tiny corner of my mind is, of course, also rejoicing in the expectation that, God willing, I will still be alive tomorrow. But it would be an egregious misrepresentation to suggest that such an expectation is the only source for the value of my life today. A patient who has experienced brain damage that prevents her from remembering the past or imagining the future might nevertheless retain the cognitive ability to enjoy the present moment. She might still enjoy the immanent physicality of eating and drinking, or the company of others, or simply being alive. The fact that she has lost the ability also to consider what the future might bring would not abolish the enjoyment she might have in the present moment, or materially affect any right she might have to continue that present enjoyment.

---

[49] Singer, *Practical Ethics*, pp. 164–65.

[50] Varner, *Personhood, ethics, and animal cognition: situating animals in Hare's two level utilitarianism*, p. 135.

Otherwise, it would presumably be morally acceptable to take life from anyone who is unaware that it is going to happen, providing it were done instantaneously and caused no suffering. Ancient Greek philosopher Epicurus was right to point out that a preference to continue to live in the future is always technically irrational because if one is alive, one is not dead, and if one is dead, one can no longer prefer to live: 'Accustom yourself to the belief that death is nothing to us. For all good and evil lie in sensation, whereas death is the privation of sensation'.[51] Even for adults, life is given inherent value by what it allows its possessor to enjoy in the moment. If futurity is not essential to biographical narrative in adults, it would be hard to argue that its absence from the capacities of childness is relevant to personal value. Killing an infant would result in the summary ending of a biographical narrative whose author is currently actively engaging with its construction and presumably enjoys doing so. Infanticide represents a harm to infants in the present moment; there is no need to define its harms by reference to the future.[52]

It is not obvious that a capacity for biographical narrative relies on a preference, or even an expectation, that life should continue into the future. On the utilitarian grounds set out here, the fact that a sense of futurity characterises adultness but not childness does not therefore provide a reason for evaluating the former more highly than the latter. A human who demonstrates only childness is capable of living and enjoying living in the present moment, whether or not he is able to hope that the enjoyment of living will continue into the future.

8.2.2.3   Autonomy

Autonomy referred to mediaeval city-states that were under the authority of the monarchy, but whose success at governing themselves meant that the monarch exempted them from the need to be directly subordinate so that they became self-governing.[53] In that original sense, the term carries not only a sense of freedom from control by others, but also the clear sense that such a freedom is contingent on habitually making the right decisions.

In contemporary medical ethics, autonomy is usually taken to represent all the cognitive abilities an individual needs in order to ensure that she is not subjected

---

[51] A. A. Long, 'Letter to Menoeceus 124', in D. N. Sedley and David Sedley (eds.), *The Hellenistic philosophers* (Cambridge: Cambridge University Press, 1987).

[52] Finnis is right to point out that infants '… can undergo unjustly inflicted harm, which damages them then and there as actual persons, even though their awareness of it as a harm and loss and impairment that they underwent may emerge in their consciousness only months or years later. Seeking … to prevent this subsequent awareness, by ensuring that the person so treated (I say harmed) is also killed before the awareness arises, no more cancels the harm in such early states or stages of an individual human person's existence than the harm is cancelled or negated or averted when an assassin ensures that his victim has no warning and no awareness of his being murdered'. Finnis, 'Capacity, harm and experience in the life of persons as equals'.

[53] "Autonomy: normative," by Mark Piper, *The Internet Encyclopedia of Philosophy*, ISSN 2161-0002, http://www.iep.utm.edu/, accessed June 2014.

against her will to invasive or intrusive interventions. That includes both the freedom to make an independent choice, and the ability to act on that choice once made. The conception of autonomy primarily as freedom from coercion arose from repugnance at discovery of the exploitation suffered by Jewish prisoners at the hands of Nazi research doctors during the Second World War. Prisoners were forced to participate in studies which often resulted in their own painful death. There was no opportunity for them to choose for themselves whether to participate or to refuse. They were treated as though they were objects that could be used as others chose to use them.

According to Beauchamp and Childress, if a patient has fully understood what a procedure entails and chooses not to allow it, then doctors are under a moral obligation not to over-ride that refusal. As we have seen, such respect for autonomy is one of the four pillars of medical ethics in Principlism.[54] Beauchamp and Childress themselves make clear that they do not consider an obligation to respect autonomy to carry any more moral weight than obligations to act fairly, do good or avoid harm. Over the years, however, it has assumed ever greater prominence in medical ethics and, of Principlism's four pillars, it is often taken by Western physicians and bioethicists to be the most important in resolving the ethical quandaries that arise in practice. Lawyer and bioethicist Carl Schneider remarks that autonomy '… has achieved paradigmatic status in both the ethics and the law of medicine' while general practitioner and moral philosopher Rana Gillon describes it as 'first among equals'.[55,56]

One result of the apotheosis of respect for autonomy in medical ethics has been that the capacities necessary to exercise it have become a measure of a patient's personal value. In clinical practice, respect for autonomy as an ethical concept is not usually disaggregated from the medico-legal understanding that persons possess undisputed ownership of their own bodies.[57] A person is protected notionally by a 'bubble', more or less coterminous with their own skin, that marks the boundary of that ownership. To allow a second person to breach the bubble, its owner must give permission. That act of permission constitutes autonomy in the context of medical interventions, and the extent to which it is given with an understanding of the

---

[54] 'The autonomous individual acts freely in accordance with a self-chosen plan, analogous to the way an independent government manages its territories and sets its policies. A person of diminished autonomy, by contrast, is in some respect controlled by others or incapable of deliberating *or acting on* the basis of his or her desires and plans'. Beauchamp and Childress, *Principles of Biomedical Ethics*, pp. 99–100 (My italics).

[55] Carl Schneider, *The practice of autonomy: patients, doctors, and medical decisions* (New York/ Oxford: Oxford University Press, 1998). In popular culture, at least in the West, it has also extended to include the idea that patients should be allowed, not only to decline interventions on the basis of their own preferences or understanding (rather than on the objectively likely benefits and harms), but also to demand treatments on the same basis.

[56] R. Gillon, 'Ethics needs principles—four can encompass the rest—and respect for autonomy should be "first among equals"', *J Med Ethics,* 29/5 (Oct 2003), 307–12.

[57] Beauchamp and Childress, *Principles of Biomedical Ethics*, p. 104.

consequences defines the term 'informed consent'.[58] The ability to reason logically about medical interventions therefore defines the legal concept of 'capacity' and, in most legislatures, the criteria for such capacity—or, more importantly, what needs to be shown in order to demonstrate that capacity is absent—are legally codified. Doctors must not proceed with an intervention without a patient's permission unless he is unable to make, and communicate, a decision for himself.[59]

It has therefore become increasingly important for doctors to distinguish carefully between patients who possess the capacities necessary to exercise it and those who do not. A duty to respect autonomy imposes on the physician an obligation to ensure interventions are not carried out in a patient who, possessing the capacity to agree to them, has chosen instead not to give permission. Under those circumstances, it would be wrong for a doctor to intervene, even if the decision she has taken will result in avoidable harm.[60] The doctor has no such obligation, however, to a patient who lacks that capacity, meaning that the property of possessing the faculties necessary to exercise autonomy in the patient determines a doctor's moral obligations towards her.[61] Doctors will act on the decision of an autonomous person because it was taken by an autonomous person, even if it is a decision that is irrational and/or will result in harm to the patient herself. If the same decision were made by someone who lacked those faculties, doctors would consider themselves under a moral obligation to over-ride it.[62] Different moral rules apply to patients labelled 'autonomous' and 'non-autonomous'. That has led some moral philosophers to ascribe to the exercise of autonomy an absolute moral value in itself; one that

---

[58] 'Informed consent' is problematic in practice. To be fully 'informed' would require not only an encyclopaedic knowledge of medicine, but also remarkable judicial skills in weighing up benefits and disbenefits of differing types and, of course, a shamanic ability to foretell the future. Furthermore, the relationship between knowledge and understanding is not straightforward. For someone with no knowledge at all, understanding is initially increased as more facts are provided. But the rate at which understanding increases diminishes as ever more facts are added. There comes a point at which a plethora of facts begins to obscure understanding rather than clarifying it; that point can be surprisingly early in the dialogue between physician and patient, however well-educated the patient may be.

[59] In the UK, the criteria for determining capacity are set out in the Mental Capacity Act (2005), Department of Health, *Mental Capacity Act (2005)* (c.9; London: HMSO, 2008).

[60] Kant's disciple, idealist philosopher Johann Fichte, points out that to claim rights against reason is nonsense. Yet people do so all the time, Fichte goes on resignedly, because: 'Man is afraid of subordinating his subjectivity to the laws of reason. He prefers tradition or arbitrariness' (Johann Gottlieb Fichte's Sämmtliche Werke, ed. I.H. Fichte (Berlin, 1846), vol. 7, 176, quoted in Berlin, *Two concepts of liberty: an inaugural lecture delivered before the University of Oxford on 31 October 1958*, p. 20).

[61] Harry G. Frankfurt, 'Freedom of the Will and the Concept of a Person', in John P. Lizza (ed.), *Defining the beginning and end of life: readings on personal identity and bioethics* (Baltimore: Johns Hopkins University Press, 2009).

[62] Under the Mental Capacity Act (2005), this would be a legal as well as a moral obligation, providing those caring for the patient—especially her family—agreed. What that means is that, paradoxically, there are circumstances under which a patient lacking capacity is more likely to receive treatment that is logically correct than the patient who possesses it.

does not depend on other personal properties and does not need to be explained by any more fundamental moral values. The capacities necessary to exercise autonomy then become a yardstick for moral value; the adjective 'autonomous' is no longer merely descriptive but has acquired de facto evaluative power. Moral philosopher John Harris, for example, considers personal value to be more or less coextensive with a capacity for autonomy: 'The point of autonomy, the point of choosing and having the freedom to choose between competing conceptions of how, and indeed why, to live, is simply that it is only thus that our lives become in any real sense our own. The value of our lives is the value we give to our lives'.[63]

There are reasons to be cautious about that evaluative power. If, for an action to be morally right, it is only necessary that the decision to act be arrived at without coercion, then there is no need for any other moral reasoning at all. As moral theologian Nigel Biggar puts it: '…the centre of gravity of Harris' account clearly lies, not in the value that we give our lives, but in the act of our giving value. Value [according to Harris] resides not in what we decide, but in that we decide. And this deciding is not responsible to anything outside of itself—it is strictly "for ourselves"; its only reason lies in the arbitrium of the individual, her arbitrary assertion'.[64] Harris' account leads quickly to a philosophical paradox: on the view he expresses, the value ('rightness') of a moral action is an expression of the extent to which it is autonomously reached. To act in a way that is morally correct, therefore, the agent's objective should be to minimise barriers to others' autonomy. But the rightness of the moral agent's action is then expressing her commitment to minimise those barriers; it does not express the extent to which the agent herself acted autonomously and so potentially contradicts the same principle if, for example, she were to decide autonomously that she does not want to minimise barriers to others' autonomy, she would be making a decision that is both morally right and wrong simultaneously.

A yardstick for personal value that links personal value ineluctably with autonomy as self-rule is doubly debilitating for childness, which encompasses neither the capacities needed to choose freely, nor those needed to act on such choices. An emphasis on the evaluative power of a capacity for autonomy, however, only succeeds in defending an adult-normative approach to personal value if the exercise of autonomy as self-rule is the only way in which an individual can construct meaningful biographical narrative. There are good reasons to think that is not the case. First, independence from the influence of others is not the only story that human beings tell about themselves. Often, it is not even an important part of that story. Humans are social creatures, and it is our relationship with other humans, rather than our freedom from their influence, that typically features most prominently in the biographical narrative we construct. Earlier we saw how even a newborn infant is capable of distinguishing between herself and other individuals. That sense of being

---

[63] Harris, 'Euthanasia and the value of life', in *Euthanasia Examined: Ethical, Clinical and Legal Perspectives*, p. 11.
[64] Nigel Biggar, *Aiming to kill: the ethics of suicide and euthanasia* (Pilgrim Press, 2004), p. 40. Author's original italics.

separate depends not only on an awareness of oneself, but also on an awareness of others. Moral philosopher Onora O'Neill points out that, despite its superficial reliance on independence from others, the concept of autonomy is in reality inherently relational because it entails acknowledging the existence and potential influence of someone other than oneself.[65] O'Neill argues that it is reasonable to extend the idea of autonomy so that it includes reliance on others within a trustful relationship.[66] Such an extension means that the range of capacities that permit autonomy is no longer restricted to those that will allow their possessor to make and act on independent decisions. Instead, it can include awareness of self in relation to others.

There is no doubt that the cognitive capacities which permit independence and agency can contribute materially to an individual's capacity for biographical narrative and can confer moral value on the terms set out here. Nor is there any doubt that those capacities are better represented in adultness than in childness. That is not enough, however, to succeed in defending the idea that an individual, and the life that he possesses, are of no value at all if he cannot make and act on independent decisions. Such a defence would require demonstration that there is only one way for an individual to construct biographical narrative, and that is to exercise self-rule, free from the influence of others. Lived experience, as well as careful reasoning, reveal that that is not true. The stories that humans tell about themselves do not always require that sort of agency or independence from others. Far from it; biographical narrative is often—perhaps usually—constructed in the context of a trustful relationship with others. Childness equips humans to construct that sort of narrative at least as well as adultness does.

8.3 Summary

Gopnik connects neurodevelopmental psychology with epistemology, but she is not promulgating a moral or philosophical theory. Her findings are a matter of observation, not ratiocination. She is presenting something that has been empirically demonstrated about what infants can do; something that is objectively true about childness. Seneca would undoubtedly have been astonished at what the twentieth and twenty-first centuries have revealed. It seems unlikely he could have imagined

---

[65] Moral philosopher Onora O'Neill points out that: '[Autonomy] is generally seen as a matter of independence, or at least as a capacity for independent decisions and action. This conception of individual autonomy sees it as relational; autonomy is always autonomy *from* something'. O'Neill, *Autonomy and trust in bioethics*, p. 23 (my italics).

[66] 'Autonomy has been a leading idea in philosophical writing on bioethics; trust has been marginal. This strikes me as surprising. Autonomy is usually identified with individual independence, and sometimes leads to ethically dubious or disastrous action. Its ethical credentials are not self-evident. Trust is surely more important, and particularly so for any ethically adequate practice of medicine, science and biotechnology. Trust–or rather loss of trust–is a constant concern in political and popular writing in all three areas' (Ibid., p. 2).

the feats of cognition of which we now know the infant human is capable at the time of birth.

Modern moral philosophy does not always seem to have kept up with the science, and the conclusions of some moral philosophers today suggest they are either unaware of the evidence, or else have chosen to ignore it. A hypothesis about infant awareness is incorrect if it relies on the idea that infants are unaware of their surroundings, or are entirely unable to process what they appreciate about those surroundings. If the infant mind is a tabula rasa, as Locke suggested, we know that it is not a tablet in the 'blank slate' sense that he may have meant it. It is much more like a tablet in the modern sense of a newly unboxed iPad.[67] It is undamaged, pristine and works perfectly. It certainly lacks the functionality of a well-used and perhaps somewhat battered older tablet, but that is not because it is incomplete, poorly made or lacks the equipment it needs to function. It is simply because the relevant apps have not yet been installed.

Evidence suggests that in fact some of the key apps are pre-installed, and that installation of others is immediate, automatic and rapid. The newborn infant is highly aware of, and engaged with, her surroundings. Bentham's casual dismissal of the infant's capacity for reasoning as less than that of a horse or a dog (*vide infra*) is no longer tenable. Even William James' more enlightened 1890 idea that the infant exists in a state of 'blooming, buzzing confusion', while prefiguring perhaps Gopnik's observations about lantern awareness, was clearly wide of the mark in characterising the infant as merely bombarded with sensations.[68] The infant is capable of love, relationships with others, pleasure experienced in the moment, such as satisfied hunger or warmth, and the capacity to invoke a caring impulse in others. She is capable of uninhibited and unfiltered perception of new sensory data, and of unbiased, though distinctively human, processing of what her senses tell her. She is, in short, perfectly capable of enjoying her existence in the present moment. Without imposing adult-normative judgements on the relative value or quality of that enjoyment, it is clear that infants, just like adults, are harmed by being killed because of what it takes from them in the present.

In the last chapter, we set out some capacities whose presence indicates that an individual is able to construct biographical narrative. Evidence shows that infants certainly have four of those: they possess the requisite anatomical equipment, they have the desire to narrate, and there are ways in which they are aware of themselves that are relevant to the construction of biographical narrative. They are born capable of relationality, considered as an awareness of other people.

The remaining two facilitators of biographical narrative from that list are reason and a sense of time passing. While a capacity for logical reason (other than a simple appreciation of the link between cause and effect) is not part of childness, there are other ways in which humans habitually reason that do not rely on such a capacity, and which very young infants can and do demonstrate. An infant has an excellent

---

[67] Other tablet analogies are available.

[68] James, *The principles of psychology.*

memory but as far as we are aware, she does not possess the capacity to imagine herself existing into the future. It is not clear, however, why the absence of such a capacity should prevent an individual from constructing biographical narrative, nor why it should be considered ethically permissible to end that construction through taking a life that is being enjoyed in the present moment.

Finally, the idea that personal value can be wholly and only expressed as the capacities necessary to exercise self-rule in isolation from the influence of others seems implausible, both on its own terms and because the exercise of autonomy in that sense is not necessary in order for humans to construct meaningful biography.

Bibliography

Agar N. How to insure against utilitarian overconfidence. Monash Bioeth Rev. 2014;32(3–4):162–71.

Akbari H, et al. Towards reconstructing intelligible speech from the human auditory cortex. Sci Rep. 2019;9(1):874.

Anand KJ, Carr DB. The neuroanatomy neurophysiology and neurochemistry of pain stress and analgesia in newborns and children. Pediatr Clin North Am. 1989;36(4):797–822.

Anand KJ, Hickey PR. Pain and its effects on the human neonate and fetus. N Engl J Med. 1987;317(21):1321–9.

Anderson JR. The development of self-recognition: a review. Dev Psychobiol. 1984;17(1):35–49.

Beauchamp T, Childress J. Principles of biomedical ethics. 6th ed. New York: Oxford University Press; 2009.

Berlin I. Two concepts of liberty: an inaugural lecture delivered before the University of Oxford on 31 October 1958. Oxford: Clarendon Press; 1958.

Biggar N. Aiming to kill: the ethics of suicide and euthanasia. Pilgrim Press; 2004.

Celano A. Medieval theories of practical reason: the thomistic doctrine of practical reason. Stanford Encyclopedia of Philosophy; 2017. https://plato.stanford.edu/entries/practical-reason-med/. Accessed 1st March.

Department of Health. Mental Capacity Act (2005), c.9. London: HMSO; 2008.

Droit-Volet S. Time perception in children: a neurodevelopmental approach. Neuropsychologia. 2013;51(2):220–34.

Farah MJ, Heberlein AS. Personhood and neuroscience: naturalizing or nihilating? Am J Bioeth. 2007;7(1):37–48.

Fonagy P, Gergely G, Target M. The parent-infant dyad and the construction of the subjective self. J Child Psychol Psychiatry. 2007;48(3–4):288–328.

Frankfurt HG. Freedom of the will and the concept of a person. In: Lizza JP, editor. Defining the beginning and end of life: readings on personal identity and bioethics. Baltimore: Johns Hopkins University Press; 2009.

Gillon R. Ethics needs principles—four can encompass the rest—and respect for autonomy should be "first among equals". J Med Ethics. 2003;29(5):307–12.

Giubilini A, Minerva F. After-birth abortion: why should the baby live? J Med Ethics. 2013;39(5):261–3.

Goksan S, et al. fMRI reveals neural activity overlap between adult and infant pain. elife. 2015;4:e06356.

Gopnik A. Why babies are more conscious than we are. Behav Brain Sci. 2007;30(5–6):503–4.

Gopnik A. The philosophical baby: what children's minds tell us about truth love & the meaning of life. London: Bodley Head; 2009.

Harris J. Euthanasia and the value of life. In: Keown J, editor. Euthanasia examined: ethical, clinical and legal perspectives. Cambridge: Cambridge University Press; 1995.

Harrison H. Whey infant surgery without anesthesia went unchallenged. New York Times, 17 Dec 1987. p. A34.

Hoffmaster B. The rationality and morality of dying children. Hast Cent Rep. 2011;41(6):30–42.

James W. The principles of psychology, Dover books on philosophy and psychology. Authorized ed. New York: Dover; 1950.

Krantz SF. Refuting Peter Singer's ethical theory: the importance of human dignity. Westport: Praeger; 2002.

Mampe B, et al. Newborns' cry melody is shaped by their native language. Curr Biol. 2009;19:1994–7.

Martin GB, Clark RD. Distress crying in neonates: species and peer specificity. Dev Psychol. 1982;18(1):3–9.

McGraw MB. Neural maturation as exemplified in the changing reactions of the infant to pin prick. Child Dev. 1941;12(1):31–42.

O'Neill O. Autonomy and trust in bioethics, Gifford lectures. Cambridge: Cambridge University Press; 2002.

Rachels J. The end of life: euthanasia and morality, Studies in bioethics. Oxford: Oxford University Press; 1986.

Rochat P. Five levels of self-awareness as they unfold early in life. Conscious Cogn. 2003;12(4):717–31.

Rochat P. The self as phenotype. Conscious Cogn. 2011;20(1):109–19.

Rochat P, Broesch T, Jayne K. Social awareness and early self-recognition. Conscious Cogn. 2012;21(3):1491–7.

Schneider C. The practice of autonomy: patients, doctors, and medical decisions. New York/ Oxford: Oxford University Press; 1998.

Singer P. Practical ethics. New York: Cambridge University Press; 2011.

Sloane A. Singer, preference utilitarianism and infanticide. Stud Christ Ethics. 1999;12(2):47–73.

Sorger B, et al. A real-time fMRI-based spelling device immediately enabling robust motor-independent communication. Curr Biol. 2012;22(14):1333–8.

Taylor C. The language animal: the full shape of the human linguistic capacity. Cambridge, MA: The Belknap Press of Harvard University Press; 2016.

Tooley M. Abortion and infanticide. Philos Public Aff. 1972;2(1):37–65.

Trevarthen C, Aitken KJ. Infant intersubjectivity: research, theory, and clinical applications. J Child Psychol Psychiatry. 2001;42(1):3–48.

Tzourio-Mazoyer N, et al. Neural correlates of woman face processing by 2-month-old infants. NeuroImage. 2002;15(2):454–61.

Varner, G.E. (2012), Personhood, ethics, and animal cognition: situating animals in Hare's two level utilitarianism (New York/Oxford: Oxford University Press).

World Health Organization. Promoting rational use of medicines: core components. In: W.H.O. policy perspectives on medicines. Geneva: World Health Organization; 2002.

Chapter 9
Changing the Orbit

Personal value, according to the way we are considering it in this book, represents the extent to which the moral agent should concern herself with an individual's interests. Since, in consequentialist terms, morally correct action represents no more than a carefully reasoned response to what the child can or cannot experience, consequentialist moral theorists can exclude very young children from such an obligation, on the grounds that childness alone does not confer on the individual a capacity to have any interests that should be relevant to the agent's moral deliberation.

Principlism objects to that conclusion and, since it commands considerable ethical authority among clinicians, it has been able to protect infants and children from the effects of consequentialist under-valuing, especially through some of its deontological claims. As long as virtually everyone agrees that the relationship between adults and children is one that imposes on the adult an obligation to be concerned with the child's interests, Principlism can accord personal value to infants and children.

As we have seen, however, that value does not flow from anything that is true about the nature of the child herself. Rather, it relies on consensus among adults regarding how adults should behave—an agreement from which many adults already dissent, and which, without a robust rational foundation, offers no guarantee of enduring in the future. It makes many of the same adult-normative assumptions that are problematic in some forms of consequentialism. It does not, for example, hold to account the assumption that an infant is cognitively incapable of enjoying her existence in the distinctively human way that is characterised by biographical narrative. It shares the belief that such a narrative is inherently valuable only to the extent that it is constructed in the manner of an ideal adult. Like Tooley and his adherents, Principlism finds itself focusing on the moral properties that an infant does *not* inherently possess, rather than proposing an anthropology based on the properties that *do* characterise an infant. Beauchamp and Childress repeatedly draw back from any conclusion that allows the lives of infants and children to be seen as less valuable than those of adults but, to those who are unconvinced by appeals to

© The Author(s), under exclusive license to Springer Nature
Switzerland AG 2026
R. Hain, *Childness and the Myth of the Unfinished Human*,
https://doi.org/10.1007/978-3-032-12111-0_9

deontological values, the reason for their discomfort is not clear, since their rejection of that conclusion does not obviously flow from a challenge to adult-normative moral thinking. The alternative account of the value of the infant and child that Principlism offers is therefore not entirely convincing. When it comes to evaluating infants and children, Principlism as it currently stands offers only a weak bulwark against adult-normative moral philosophical thinking.

9.1 Principlism Through an Age-Neutral Lens

Principlism does not set out to be universalisable in the way that a single coherent moral theory would. In contrast with, say, Kant's claims for deontology or Bentham's for utilitarian consequentialism, the principles it offers do not claim to be equally valid in all circumstances. Quite the opposite; physician philosopher Raanan Gillon points out that, if Principlism is to inform correct behaviour in respect of patients, it must be carefully contextualised. Its principles need to be specified to the moral quandary under consideration, a process Gillon describes as paying 'attention to scope' and which he considers to be as important to Principlism as any of the principles themselves.[1]

The task of specifying a principle is the task of identifying the more fundamental values that underlie it, and on that basis considering how it should inform the ethical question at hand. If we are to reject adult-normative moral reasoning in favour of reasoning that is age-neutral, the challenge is to specify Principlism to children—attending appropriately to its scope, as Gillon might put it. There are ways in which human children are more similar to one another than they are to adult humans and vice versa. Even if the differences between childness and adultness do not justify evaluating one more highly than the other, some of them must be germane to moral reasoning.

The aim of specifying Principlism to children is not to suggest that we should consider childness rather than adultness to be normative for all humans. That would substitute one unjustified prejudice for another. Specifying the principles to children means showing how the more fundamental values from which the principles flow can manifest in an individual who possesses only childness. It does not entail dismissing any of the principles altogether, but is rather that of imagining what each would look like if it were viewed, not through the usual adult-normative lens, but through an age-neutral one; a perspective that consciously gives the same value to the cognitive characteristics of childness as it does to those of adultness.

---

[1] R. Gillon, 'Medical ethics: four principles plus attention to scope', *British Medical Journal,* 309 (1994), 184–88.

9.1.1   Interests

Earlier we identified three important practical problems in establishing interests in infants and children. The first is that the capacities of childness mean that an infant appreciates her existence and that of the universe in a way that does not rely on characteristics of adultness such as logical reason, independence from others or an understanding of the future. An age-neutral approach acknowledges that there may be many ways in which an individual can construct a meaningful biographical narrative in the here and now. Enjoyment of one's existence in a distinctively human way does not rely exclusively on capacities that an infant lacks and so, on the age-neutral view, the infant's experience of being alive and appreciating the world in the present moment is enough on its own to constitute an interest.

The intersubjective nature of a child's normal existence means her interests may not be separable from those of others, especially her family. While most would not express it in that way, there is a sense in which some parents intuitively expect to have the same rights over an infant as they would over a possession. If that were true, any benefits to the infant would not merely be *described* by her parents but would actually be *defined* by them. When speaking for a child using the voice of an owner, parents would effectively be speaking for themselves. What is right or wrong is for the child would be determined wholly in the arbitrium of parental preferences; even though the person most affected is the child, a medical decision would be morally right in the same fact that it is what her parents prefer. Their preferences for the child would simply express their own interests, and they would make medical decisions in the same way that they might choose whether or not to take on or continue with the inconvenient tasks associated with keeping a guinea-pig or a washing-machine.[2] We have seen that ideas of parental ownership have persisted, albeit in a weak form, into the twenty-first century.[3] On the face of it, an age-neutral approach to ethics requires that when a doctor is considering a medical decision in a child the interests of adults—even the child's parents—must be excluded from consideration under the principles of beneficence and non-maleficence, because they are not the interests of the patient in question. If we accept that the way in which infants participate in their own biographical narrative is no less valid for inherent value than the way adults do so, then it is clear that the infant has interests of her own and we must emphatically reject the idea that an adult is permitted to identify a child's interests wholly with her own. On age-neutral terms she cannot possess a child, any more than she could possess another adult.

---

[2] The extreme utilitarian view represented by Singer is that parents of an infant need speak in no other mode than as the infant's owner. Dominic Wilkinson, a philosopher who is also a practising neonatologist, acknowledges that even an infant might have interests in her own right although he suggests they can be offset by the interests of her parents: 'The crucial question' he says 'is *how much weight* parents' interests should be given relative to the interests of the child?' Dominic Wilkinson, *Death or disability?: the 'Carmentis machine' and decision-making for critically ill children* (Oxford: Oxford University Press, 2013), p. 2.

[3] Birchley, 'Charlie Gard and the weight of parental rights to seek experimental treatment'.

But that does not entail that a child's family's interests can be set aside as though they were entirely irrelevant. It is not always possible wholly to disentangle the interests of an infant from those of her parents because the infant herself does not see her own interests as separate from those of others. A child might easily agree to an intervention that is of no medical value, because he knows that is what his mother wants. That need not represent exploitation, because, using an appropriately capacious understanding of a child's interests, a preference for obeying his mother should be made part of the calculus of the child's own interests. An age-neutral approach to medical ethics underlines the fact that in making medical decisions doctors might have to consider interests to be important and relevant without being able to annexe them exclusively to the child herself. The doctor must consider the interests of a dyad of child and adult, which may be neither wholly those of the child, nor wholly those of the adult.[4]

Another challenge that age-neutrality offers to the principles of beneficence and non-maleficence is that the interests of an infant or child are relevant to moral deliberation even if they are not clearly knowable. On the age-neutral view, in weighing a child's interests, it is not enough to consider objective facts about him, such as what her oxygen levels are or whether he has a chest infection. We also need to consider what his own subjective experience of his existence might be. A child's subjective judgement of what constitutes 'well-being' is relevant to an assessment of benefits and harms, because a rational understanding of well-being must take account of the individual's own experience, including his or her perception of what matters. A child with cancer, for example, might choose not to take regular analgesic medication because she does not want her friends to think she is an addict, even though the result is that she experiences physical pain that is, in fact, unnecessary and avoidable. Her choice to experience physical pain is not necessarily a 'bad' choice. It is a rational one that balances the relative impacts of pain and social stigma on that individual's well-being. The moral agent who seeks to act in the best interests of a child needs to know something about what that child is currently experiencing, and what he will experience as a result of the agent's decision; his understanding of sociality and relationships, his likes and dislikes or his preferences about treatments.

It is the nature of childness to be unable to express subjective preferences verbally and, although with the passage of time he will become increasingly sophisticated in his ability to formulate and communicate his preferences, it will be well

---

[4]That is not quite the same as saying that there are circumstances under which the interests of a child's family should be weighed against the interests of the child. That sort of weighing would still require interests to be resolved and annexed to individuals. In *Best Interests and the Carmentis Machine*, Dominic Wilkinson makes a utilitarian argument for weighing the interests of an infant against those of her parents and even those of other infants Wilkinson, *Death or disability?: the 'Carmentis machine' and decision-making for critically ill children*. While Wilkinson does not challenge the idea that interests can be annexed to an individual, his approach is practical and such a calculus among individual interests would logically usually result in the same conclusion as one based on an intersubjective account of interests, at least to the extent that unknowable interests are correctly inferred.

into teenage before his capacity to do so approaches that of an adult. On the age-neutral view, however, we should not fail to take into account an infant or child's own experience just because it is difficult to know, because that would inappropriately restrict our ideas about her well-being. Subjective interests are difficult to assess objectively; they exist only as an individual's subjective perceptions. They nevertheless represent facts about her that are relevant to her biographical narrative and so represent interests that need to be considered. If we dismiss an infant or child's own experience of the world because we consider it to be irrelevant to meaningful biographical narrative, we will inevitably consider her 'well-being' in a way that is importantly incomplete. Her subjective interests cannot be known with certainty, but the obligation of adults towards infants and children cannot be that they only act on certainty; rather, it is that they act in a child's interests to the extent that they are able to do so.

The doctor might also need to consider the interests of parents. A doctor has a duty of obligatory beneficence to other people, irrespective of their age. Taking an age-neutral position does not negate that duty, or imply that it can be restricted to attending only to a specific child's interest, even for a paediatrician. The argument here has been that the way infants and children experience the world is no less valuable, considered as a source of human well-being, than the way adults experience it. It certainly does not entail that adultness is consistently *less* valuable in that sense than childness is. What that means in practice is that a doctor must consider parents' preferences to be morally relevant interests in themselves.

Viewing the principles of beneficence and non-maleficence through an age-neutral lens extends them in three important ways. It expands the way in which the moral agent should conceive benefits and harms (interests) so that it includes modes of enjoying existence that are more inchoate than logical reason or futurity but are nevertheless inherently valuable in their own right. It acknowledges that individuals exist in relationship with others, and that sometimes such a relationship is so close that it is impossible to separate the interests of the individual parties in order to weigh them against one another. And it acknowledges too that there are some harms and benefits relevant to moral deliberation that need to be considered by an agent, even though they cannot be known with certainty. Under those circumstances, the agent is under an obligation to infer as closely as possible what those harms and benefits are, which usually means dialogue with those who know the individual best.

Such an extension of how interests are conceived extends the scope of Principlism to infants and children, because it does not reference adultness but is explained by, and so accords inherent value to, childness.

9.1.2 Respect for Autonomy

In Principlism, the emphasis of autonomy is on voluntariness. The capacities that make an individual autonomous are those that permit ' … self-rule that is free from both controlling interference by others and from limitations, such as inadequate understanding, that prevent meaningful choice' and allow her to '… act freely in accordance with a self-chosen plan'.[5] At a stretch, we might consider that there is a sense in which even very young children can be said to possess such a capacity.[6] We saw earlier that autonomy, considered as self-rule, does not depend simply on the cognitive abilities of an individual person alone, but is also influenced by the complexity and seriousness of the decision. A child's capacity to exercise autonomy could therefore be said to depend on the question she is being asked, as well as on her cognitive abilities. A certain 2-year-old is unlikely to be able to demonstrate autonomy by agreeing to treatment for leukaemia, but that same child would nevertheless be able to demonstrate it by agreeing to have a sticking plaster on a minor cut.

Accepting that some children can and should make some medical decisions autonomously does not represent an age-neutral perspective, however, because in those cases a child is not deploying the capacities of childness, but rather the rational capacities of adultness that he has already acquired.[7] It appeals to the same conception of autonomy as self-rule that characterises adult-normative thinking in medical ethics. If childness permits any kind of autonomy at all, it must be of a kind that is different from what constitutes autonomy in adults.[8] According to an age-neutral approach, the concept of autonomy is not exhausted by whether or not an individual is independent of others, or possesses the cognitive capabilities necessary to give informed consent. It is the infant's dependence on others, rather than her independence from them, that is a central plank of the biographical narrative she constructs. Decisions that impact the infant's own interests inevitably arise in a relational context that includes others in the universe, rather than being in isolation from them.

---

[5] Beauchamp and Childress, *Principles of Biomedical Ethics*, pp. 99–100.

[6] Paediatrician and ethicist Paul Baines proposes actively supporting a child's development of the 'adult' capacities necessary to exercise autonomy: 'Children do not suddenly, overnight, develop the abilities which are needed for a person to act autonomously. A child's ability to act autonomously will mature if the child is encouraged to develop the abilities which underlie her competence to make autonomous decisions. Perhaps a child should be encouraged to take responsibility, at first in areas where the consequences of choosing unwisely are less severe or are short term' (Baines, 'Medical ethics for children: applying the four principles to paediatrics'). Article 5 of the UN Convention on the Rights of the Child demands that states respect the 'evolving capacities of the child' (United Nations General Assembly, *Convention on the Rights of the Child: adopted and opened for signature, ratification and accession by General Assembly resolution 44/25*) and some form of graduated approach to autonomy is accommodated in many legislatures.

[7] Cristina Traina suggests that, in older children, a lack of autonomy is explained by restrictions imposed by her size and the extent to which children are culturally prevented from influencing others in society. Such essentially practical limitations on autonomy say little about the child's own capacity for moral awareness, deliberation or choice, and nothing substantive about whether a child is capable of moral agency: '… development is incidental to … standing as a dignified moral agent'. Cristina L. H. Traina, 'Children and moral agency', *Journal of the Society of Christian Ethics*, 29/2 (Winter/Fall 2009), 19–37.

[8] Neil C. Manson and Onora O'Neill, *Rethinking informed consent in bioethics* (Cambridge: Cambridge University Press, 2007).

Principlism already makes the general observation that doctors are wrong to assume that an obligation to respect autonomy means they must insist patients make medical decisions themselves. The risk is that a duty to help the patient towards restoration of health in accordance with the principles of beneficence and non-maleficence becomes secondary to a perceived duty to avoid making decisions, in accordance with what the principle of respect for autonomy seems to demand.[9] Patients find themselves always unable to delegate decisions, *even if they want to.* Beauchamp and Childress rightly point out that such an understanding inverts the roles of moral agent and moral patient in the relationship from which the duty flows: 'Autonomous choice is a *right*—not a *duty*—of patients'.[10] In other words, according to Principlism, physicians must certainly respect autonomy in patients who possess it, but there is no reciprocal obligation on patients to be autonomous, even if they can. The concept that Principlism references here is that of trust; the idea that it must be open to individuals to leave decision-making to others, even where the individual possesses the necessary cognitive capacities to make the decision herself.[11] In practice, that is what happens in real life. Real persons exist in a web of relationships, whatever their age, and a decision made by any normally functioning person will be influenced by those relationships. Even adults usually exercise autonomy in a context that includes, and indeed may be defined by, the influence of other people, and a concept of autonomy that identifies it exclusively with a capacity for self-rule is perhaps of more limited relevance to medical ethics in practice than is currently often assumed, even when it comes to medical decisions that might prolong life or allow death to supervene.[12]

---

[9] It should be noted that there are many, especially outside the Western ethical traditions, who have little patience for the idea that there is absolute moral value in autonomy, even in adults. Turkish bioethicist Jukka Varelius comments that: '… where autonomous patients want to make choices that they admit to be bad for them, it is more plausible to take them to be speaking about "badness" in inverted commas than to accept that there is intrinsic value in autonomy that could overweigh the harm or loss of wellbeing that they would suffer as a result of their making bad choices'. J. Varelius, 'The value of autonomy in medical ethics', *Med Health Care Philos,* 9/3 (2006), 377–88. See also Council of Europe, *Convention for the Protection of Human Rights and Dignity of the Human Being with regard to the Application of Biology and Medicine: Convention on Human Rights and Biomedicine, Oviedo, 4.IV.1997* (Strasbourg: Council of Europe, 1997).

[10] Beauchamp and Childress, *Principles of Biomedical Ethics,* p. 107. (authors' italics).

[11] Jukka Varelius argues on consequentialist grounds that if individual autonomy is seen as a procedural insistence on making decisions outwith the influence of others, it represents no more than a failure to delegate decision-making. That failure is irrational if the individual fails to delegate to those who are more likely than herself to make a choice that is, in fact, in her best interests, or more likely to result in what she desires. Such an irrational failure to trust others, Varelius suggests, restricts rather than facilitating autonomy. 'Indeed, if others are more capable of getting the kind of results that the person wants, the person who lets others make her choices for her can thereby become even more autonomous than she were to begin with. This is because, as a consequence of letting others make her important choices for her, her life goes more in the way that she wants than it would have gone if she had made her choices by herself'. Varelius, 'The value of autonomy in medical ethics', p. 383.

[12] '[i]n the field of the choice between life and death therefore, resort to the notion of individual autonomy is in part an illusion. [A] patient [whose physical and mental faculties are deteriorating]

Onora O'Neill points out that there is a sense in which the whole concept of autonomy as freedom from influence by others is paradoxical because identifying oneself as an individual at all entails prior awareness of a relationship with others. The concept of separateness logically requires a prior concept of relationship; in a universe that contained only one being, that being would have no concept of itself as 'separate' until another being appeared for it to see itself, as it were, as 'separate from'. O'Neill proposes that meaningful autonomy need not, in fact, express isolation from the influence of others, but rather can express the relationship between individuals. An individual can express meaningful autonomy by choosing to allow someone else to decide; in other words, by trusting them to act in her interest. Individual autonomy in that sense can be said to be 'intersubjective'; that is, characterising a relationship between individuals rather than demanding isolation from such relationships.[13] In achieving desirable outcomes in bioethics, O'Neill suggests that such trust in others has a more reliable track record than procedural conceptions of autonomy that rely on independence.[14] If autonomy can manifest as trust in others, as O'Neill suggests, then individuals can express autonomy even if they are not obviously capable of self-rule. Someone can meaningfully express autonomy, even if the only procedural criterion for autonomy they are able to demonstrate is a capacity to delegate decisions.

That sets the bar for individual autonomy very low: perhaps low enough to be leapt by an infant. On age-neutral terms, one reason that adults are entitled to make medical decisions over a child is to suggest that there is some de facto way in which the infant or child can meaningfully be said to have delegated authority to her parents. The claim for trust as a form of autonomy is that an individual can demonstrate it by delegating decision-making to another person. One of the defining characteristics of an infant is dependence on others, and the moral authority of parents to make decisions on behalf of their child could be characterised as an example (albeit extreme) of a patient demonstrating autonomy of that relational sort. One objection might be that the child is not delegating in any meaningful sense because she is not making a conscious decision to trust someone else. But that would return us to narrow and adult-normative conceptions of reason as exclusively a matter of logic, and of autonomy as exclusively a matter of self-rule. It is part of the dependent and

---

may truly want to die, but this desire is not the fruit of his freedom alone. It may be—and most often is—the translation of the attitude of those around him, if not of society as a whole which no longer believes in the Value of his life and signals this to him in all sorts of ways. Here we have a supreme paradox: someone is cast out of the land of the living and then thinks that he, personally, wants to die'. Emmanuel Hirsch (1986) quoted and translated by Nigel Biggar Biggar, *Aiming to kill: the ethics of suicide and euthanasia*, p. 138.

[13] 'This conception of individual autonomy sees it as *intersubjective:* autonomy is always autonomy from something; as *selective:* individuals may be independent in some matters but not in others; and as *graduated:* some individuals may have greater and others lesser degrees of independence'. O'Neill, *Autonomy and trust in bioethics*, p. 23.

[14] 'Autonomy has been a leading idea in philosophical writing on bioethics; trust has been marginal. This strikes me as surprising. Autonomy is usually identified with individual independence, and sometimes leads to ethically dubious or disastrous action. Its ethical credentials are not self-evident. Trust is surely more important, and particularly so for any ethically adequate practice of medicine, science and biotechnology' (Ibid., p. ix).

trustful nature of an infant or child to leave important decisions to someone else. He assumes that those around him will make decisions on his behalf; he is exercising a form of relational autonomy by instinctively trusting the adults around him. There is a sense, in other words, in which a physician respects a child's autonomy by acknowledging that one characteristic of childness is to trust a parent.

On the age-neutral view, a capacity to acknowledge one's dependence on others and to be willing to delegate decision-making is as valuable a part of the normal human's experience of the world as the capacities that are necessary to take decisions independently of others' influence. Again, broadening how autonomy is conceived beyond self-rule to encompass trust and interdependence accords inherent value to childness and extends the scope of Principlism to infants and children.

9.1.3 Justice

In healthcare, justice is usually taken to refer to a fair distribution of resources by society. The ethical demand that justice-as-fairness makes of clinicians is an obligation to ensure that financial resources are used in a way that maximises the benefit to all those who are entitled to benefit from them. If resources are finite, then the demands of justice-as-fairness must inevitably restrict what should be made available to any one individual patient. The extent of that restriction depends on the number of those who are entitled to benefit and among whom resources are to be shared. The principle of justice as fairness therefore critically depends on defining the population of beings to whom ideas of fairness should apply; that is, society.

Adult-normative ideas of society in Principlism rely, as we have seen, on contractarian ideas of reciprocity between its members that are problematic in children. The concept of reciprocity is antithetical to the dependent character of childness. Infants depend on adults, but there is no 'two-way street'; adults in society do not depend on infants (except perhaps in the broadest sense that continuation of the human race relies on their existence). Reciprocity requires a capacity for altruism, which in turn requires reasoning capacities that childness does not encompass.

An adult-normative account of justice starts with the observation 'This is society' and goes on to ask the question, 'Is an infant the sort of human who should be considered part of it?' That already pre-supposes that there is something inherent about the infant that casts some doubt over her participation. We have seen how Engelhardt, for example, defines society on the basis of reciprocal moral agency and so finds himself compelled to exclude infants because they do not have moral agency.

Physician philosopher Sjoren Holm argues that, logically, a definition of society should flow from the most inclusive way of describing those who are in it, rather than from some antecedent set of criteria such as Engelhardt's insistence on moral agency.[15] If we set adult-normative assumptions about the nature of society aside,

---

[15] Holm, 'The peaceable pluralistic society and the question of persons', p. 385. Holm's reasoning is that Engelhardt is wrong to identify personhood exclusively with moral agency, because a normative definition of personhood can be rationally reached among individuals who are entirely

the initial observation is: 'This is an individual who exhibits only childness' and the follow-up question becomes, 'What would a society look like if it valued childness and adultness equally ?' Infants are already members of society; the question, as Holm sees it, is how to define society in a way that explains their membership. Rawls' exclusion of children from the ideal society comes from his low opinion of their ability to understand the needs of others, an opinion which draws heavily on the psychological theories of Rousseau and Piaget.[16] We now know that there is no age at which a child is entirely unaware of the beliefs, intentions, and feelings of others. Alison Gopnik goes further and suggests that it is childness, rather than adultness, that is most likely to avoid the perils of abstraction in the way we treat others in society. A willingness to categorise others as less valuable because they are different, for example, is more characteristic of adultness than childness.[17] Moral theologian Stanley Hauerwas points out that society itself relies on, and is to a certain extent defined by, 'trustful relationships'.[18] On that basis, Hauerwas considers that 'children, even infants, can have a moral role in the community'.[19] As we have seen, trust is a skill for which childness naturally equips individuals—perhaps rather better than adultness does. Developing the infant's natural gift for trust, and ensuring it survives the ravages of adultness, is the task that society delegates to a child's family.[20]

An age-neutral view, by acknowledging that the notion of society articulates a concept of interdependence rather than simple reciprocity, allows for the possibility that there might be ways in which an infant can be considered to participate in society even without a capacity for adult-type reason. Viewing the principle of justice through an age-neutral lens represents society as a social construct that describes relationships between people, rather than just a rather complex vehicle for quid pro quo. That conception of society accords value to the kind of intersubjective skills that

---

dependent on others and therefore cannot participate in society if it is considered only as a reciprocal moral project.

[16] 'The child has not yet mastered the art of perceiving the person of others, that is, the art of discerning their beliefs, intentions, and feelings, so that an awareness of these things cannot inform his interpretation of their behavior. Moreover, his ability to put himself in their place is still untutored and likely to lead him astray. It is no surprise, then, that these elements, so important from the final moral point of view, are left out of account at the earliest stage ...' Rawls, *A Theory of Justice*, p. 411 Sect 71.

[17] 'Often a return to the intimate empathy of infancy—that immediate sense of how other people feel—can be the most powerful way to change what people do. For example, we dehumanize people in the "out-group"—people who are not like us. This impulse is deep-seated and very difficult to overturn completely. One of the best ways to change it is to actually become intimate with the out-group—to recognize that those people are actually like me'. Gopnik, *The Philosophical Baby*, p. 231.

[18] S. Hauerwas, *Suffering presence* (Notre Dame: University of Notre Dame Press, 1986), p. 132.

[19] Ibid., p. 138.

[20] The view that teaching children to be 'other-centred' is a primary task of parenthood is supported by empirical psychological research. D. Baumrind, 'Parental discipline and social competence in children', *Youth and Society*, 9 (1978), 238–76.

childness does encompass, as well as the sort of moral reasoning skills that it does not. If society is viewed in an age-neutral manner, humans can participate in society *because of* the characteristics of childness, not *in spite* of them. This perspective extends the scope of justice-as-fairness in Principlism to include infants and children.

9.2 Summary

The exercise of considering how each of its principles might change when Principlism is viewed through an age-neutral lens represents the process of specification that Gillon considers so important to Principlism's validity. It enables us to see what Principlism would look like if it started with the assumption that the cognitive characteristics of childness are as valid for meaningful existence as those of adultness.

An age-neutral approach gives the same value to the contribution made to biographical narrative by immediate sensation and existence as it does to that of memories of the past or expectations of the future, and recognises that it can be important to consider the interests of a relational dyad or triad without being able to resolve them unequivocally into the interests of component individuals. It insists that interests may be morally relevant and important without always being expressible by the patient or precisely knowable by the moral agent.

An age-neutral approach extends the concept of respect for autonomy from insisting on self-rule, isolated from the influence of others, to the idea of supporting decisions in a context of networks of relationships. Ultimately, that leads to the idea of trust; the notion that there are relationships in which the most appropriate decision-maker is not the individual patient, but someone to whom he has implicitly or explicitly delegated authority to make decisions. On age-neutral terms, the infant can be treated as though they were capable of trust because that is the normal mode in which an infant relates to others. Finally, an age-neutral approach makes clear that the intersubjective and relational capacities that characterise childness can equip an individual for participation in the community project that constitutes society, and that infants and children are part of society because they are already part of the network of relationships and community that a society comprises. If society is defined in such a way as to exclude individuals who possess only the cognitive skills of childness, it is not because infants and children lack important capacities, but because it is an adult-normative definition of society that is too restricted.

Bibliography

Baines P. Medical ethics for children: applying the four principles to paediatrics. J Med Ethics. 2008;34(3):141–5.
Baumrind D. Parental discipline and social competence in children. Youth Soc. 1978;9:238–76.

Beauchamp T, Childress J. Principles of biomedical ethics. 6th ed. New York: Oxford University Press; 2009.

Biggar N. Aiming to kill: the ethics of suicide and euthanasia. Pilgrim Press; 2004.

Birchley G. Charlie Gard and the weight of parental rights to seek experimental treatment. J Med Ethics. 2018;44(7):448–52.

Council of Europe. Convention for the protection of human rights and dignity of the human being with regard to the application of biology and medicine: convention on human rights and biomedicine, Oviedo, 4.IV.1997. Strasbourg: Council of Europe; 1997.

Gillon R. Medical ethics: four principles plus attention to scope. Br Med J. 1994;309:184–8.

Gopnik A. The philosophical baby: what children's minds tell us about truth love & the meaning of life. London: Bodley Head; 2009.

Hauerwas S. Suffering presence. Notre Dame: University of Notre Dame Press; 1986.

Holm S. The peaceable pluralistic society and the question of persons. J Med Philos. 1988;13(4):379–86.

Manson NC, O'Neill O. Rethinking informed consent in bioethics. Cambridge: Cambridge University Press; 2007.

Mullin A. Children and the argument from 'marginal' cases. Ethical Theory Moral Pract. 2011;14(3):291–305.

O'Neill O. Autonomy and trust in bioethics, Gifford lectures. Cambridge: Cambridge University Press; 2002.

Rawls J. A theory of justice. Cambridge, MA: Belknap Press of Harvard University Press; 1999.

Traina CLH. Children and moral agency. J Soc Christ Ethics. 2009;29(2):19–37.

Varelius J. The value of autonomy in medical ethics. Med Health Care Philos. 2006;9(3):377–88.

Wilkinson, D. (2013), Death or disability?: the 'Carmentis machine' and decision-making for critically ill children (Oxford: Oxford University Press).

Chapter 10
The Cognitively Impaired Child

So far in this book I have focused on childness considered as a normal mode in which humans habitually appreciate and engage with the universe. In practice, however, that is not the context in which the most ethically challenging decisions concerning children are typically made. Ethical quandaries are often the result of an illness that threatens to bring to a premature end the life of a child whose cognition is not normal, but is impaired, either because she has suffered brain damage or is seriously unwell, or both.

There are non-consequentialist values that can explain the obligations of a doctor to such a child because they do not depend on the capacity of the individual to benefit. Doctors are, for example, expected to treat patients in a way that respects their dignity. That expectation is not connected to the capacity of a particular patient to benefit from respectful treatment. An obligation to respect dignity might even extend to patients who have died. The medical student who shows consideration to the cadaver she is dissecting is offering no benefit to the cadaver, but there is a sense in which the cadaver remains human, and so deserves some of the respect due to humans, because other humans relate to it as such.[1] The cadaver does not care how it is treated, but when deciding to treat the cadaver as though it did care—in other words, to treat it with dignity—the student's moral reasoning is shaped by an understanding of the needs and perceptions of humanity in general and the fact that, in

---

[1] Professor of clinical anatomy and theological ethicist D. Gareth Jones locates the importance of such respect in a theology of the physical body: 'Respect for the dead body now foreshadows respect for the resurrection body in the future. Consequently, any willingness to desecrate or devalue the dead body shows a disregard for what that person may become, alongside a disregard for what that person has been … our bodies constitute the one common strand between what we are now and what we may become' (D. Gareth Jones, 'The dead body as an object of investigation', in John J. Fitzgerald and Ashley John Moyse (eds.), *Treating the body in medicine and religion: Jewish, Christian, and Islamic perspectives* (1st edn.; London: Routledge, 2018), p. 202).

R. Hain, *Childness and the Myth of the Unfinished Human*,
https://doi.org/10.1007/978-3-032-12111-0_10

practice, persons identify themselves in relation to other persons who feature in their story, alive or dead.[2]

It seems clear that on those grounds such an obligation must also extend to children who are so damaged that they can derive no personal benefit from being treated well. If someone can and should be treated with respect even after they have died, it would be difficult to deny that the same is true of a child who is still alive, even if she herself is unaware of being treated well. The way in which a doctor should care for her might be important for reasons that have nothing to do with the capacities of the individual patient (though, in passing, they might have a lot to do with the character of the doctor).

The vast majority of children whose cognition is impaired, however, do not fall into the same unaware category as a cadaver, and we do not have to rely on non-consequentialist values in order to explain why an agent should concern herself with the interests of a child with cognitive impairment. The extent to which damage to the brain impacts a child's awareness is highly variable, and the range of ways in which an infant or child might be harmed is very wide. Triangulating through both, there is no doubt that there are actions that an agent can take that will harm a child with cognitive impairment, and there is no doubt either that the child herself is often aware that such harm is taking place. A child who is unable to reason logically or to contemplate the future, for example, might nevertheless be capable of experiencing (and, *pace* Sidgwick and Kuhse, being aware of the fact that she is experiencing) pain or other modes of suffering in the present moment. Even on the most restrictive of consequentialist terms, such children possess some inherent value because their cognition means they are capable of benefiting from actions that are morally correct and being harmed by those that are morally wrong.

Those consequentialist terms, however, leave open the possibility that the inherent value of a child whose cognition is impaired might be less than that of a child whose brain is undamaged. There are many clinical situations in which that hierarchy of value might be brought into contention. Perhaps the commonest is when it comes to her consumption of intensive care resources. If a child is admitted to intensive care, it is usually in order to have invasive ventilation. Its objective is to support breathing for a matter of a few days or weeks while the child's body recovers from a serious acute illness. A plastic airway is inserted into his airway and attached to an artificial ventilator. The procedure is harmful, in the sense that it is painful and uncomfortable for the child and because the presence of the tube and the pressure of the ventilated gases cause physical damage to the respiratory system. But, by ensuring enough oxygen gets into the blood and enough carbon dioxide gets out, invasive ventilation buys enough time for the seriously unwell child to heal, and, by doing

---

[2]Anthropologist Greg Dening takes the same idea further when he considers the dignity of the 'voiceless dead' in interpretations of history (Greg Dening, 'Giving the Past Its Dignity', in Jeff Malpas and Norelle Lickiss (eds.), *Perspectives on human dignity: a conversation. 1* (Dordrecht: Springer, 2007). Again, dignity here refers to the idea that there are people who cannot themselves benefit from being treated well, but whom Dening argues should be treated as though they can for the sake of other humans.

so, can help restore a child to full health. The harms are real and significant, but they are short-term and easily justified by the clear benefits of keeping a child alive while healing takes place.

Over recent decades, the proportion of children being admitted to intensive care who are cognitively impaired has risen inexorably.[3] Rather than an acute infection or serious injury from which, given time and ventilatory support, they will recover, nowadays it is common for children to be admitted to intensive care because they have experienced an acute respiratory complication of some underlying neurological condition that is progressive and incurable. The nature of their condition means that they are likely to remain in the intensive care unit for many weeks or months, and there is no prospect of a return to ways of appreciating their existence that would be usual for other children of their age.[4] The change has been a difficult one for paediatric intensivists to navigate. In the past, intensive care was a career that involved developing a high degree of skill in carrying out technically sophisticated life-saving interventions in acutely unwell children in a tightly controlled environment. The interventions were painful and sometimes dangerous, but their harms were easily justified by their potential to restore a child to the sort of existence usual for someone of that age. Today, many intensivists find themselves instead ventilating the same child time after time over a period of some years, each chest infection more serious than the last, each recovery taking longer than the one before and permitting a return to a baseline level of health that declines steadily with every episode.

Sometimes, there is no prospect of returning even to a level of health that would allow the child to breathe independently. For any child with a rapidly progressive neurological condition, there comes a point at which the brain is no longer able to maintain breathing. If that occurs while the child is already being ventilated, as it often does, discontinuing ventilation makes it highly likely that the child will die.[5] Intensivists find themselves in an even more difficult position once it is clear that the child has reached that point. The benefits of continuing ventilation are now illusory or at best speculative, while the harms of doing so are ongoing and certain. For most children under those circumstances, there is little doubt that it would be better for the child if ventilation were discontinued. Under a variety of motivating influences, however, including the process of grieving that they themselves are having to go through, parents sometimes request that invasive ventilation be continued. Even in countries where the law does not require doctors to act in accordance with that

---

[3] J. E. Rennick and J. E. Childerhose, 'Redefining success in the PICU: new patient populations shift targets of care', *Pediatrics,* 135/2 (Feb 2015), e289–91.

[4] Adrian Plunkett and Roger C. Parslow, 'Is it taking longer to die in paediatric intensive care in England and Wales?', *Archives of Disease in Childhood,* 101/9 (2016).

[5] It is important to distinguish this carefully from 'brain death', which is legally defined. While there is some inconsistency across different legislatures, in most the term describes a much greater degree of cognitive impairment than is usually the case at the time discontinuation of invasive ventilation is mooted. A. McGee and D. Gardiner, 'Differences in the definition of brain death and their legal impact on intensive care practice', *Anaesthesia,* 74/5 (2019), 569–72.

request, most would find it difficult in practice to go against the wishes of a parent, especially one who is faced with the anguish of losing a child.

Furthermore, paediatric intensivists are constantly aware that at any time they might be called on to save the life of another child whose cognition is not impaired, and that if all the beds in one intensive care unit are occupied, the doctor will be forced to send a critically injured child on a long and perhaps perilous journey to another unit that might be many miles away. Many have come to see themselves as guardians of a scarce resource, and to feel it is their responsibility to weigh the interests of the actual cognitively impaired child in front of them today against those of the hypothetical child who might get hit by a car tomorrow and who could be returned to a normal life if only a bed were to remain available. The intensivist is therefore in an invidious position; in order to attend to the interests of a child's parents, he or she feels under pressure to act in respect of the child in a way that not only represents a net harm to that patient, but might simultaneously put at risk the lives of other patients, as yet hypothetical.

10.1   Value and Valuing

Against that background, it is understandable that there is an appetite for defining a category of child to whom the paraphernalia of intensive care should simply not be made available. At a national conference for paediatricians in the UK some years ago, one speaker suggested to a large audience of paediatric delegates that cognitively impaired children should properly be considered no more persons than some non-human primates, and that expensive intensive care facilities should not be provided for them for that reason.[6]

The conference audience was troubled by the speaker's apparent willingness to ascribe different values to children on the basis of their cognitive abilities. At the same time, most people in the audience agreed that there are certain specific children who should not be ventilated, and even agreed that cognitive impairment might be the reason. The two responses represent two ways of evaluating the child that are superficially similar but in reality are quite distinct. The speaker's concern was to define the sort of patient who need not be the object of a doctor's concern. His claim was that if a child's cognitive function is sufficiently low, the patient is not, as it were, 'one of us' and the doctor, as a moral agent, need not concern herself with that child's interests at all. Such a child should not be ventilated, the speaker suggested, because her cognitive impairment consigns her to a category of children whose personal value is less than that of other children. The audience, on the other hand,

---

[6]The obvious retort here is that without reference to the benefits and harms ventilation might offer, the speaker's logic argues just as strongly that we should ventilate non-human primates. The speaker invoked Peter Singer, but there is a sense in which his reasoning was entirely at odds with that of Singer, who explicitly rejects the idea that individuals should be treated on the basis of their membership of a certain category or species. See Singer, *Practical Ethics*, p. 68.

insisted that the value of a child whose cognition is impaired is exactly the same as any other child's. The doctor's response to that value is to concern herself with the child's interests, just as she would for any other child, and in doing so to ask the question "In what should my concern consist, bearing in mind the circumstances of this particular child?" A child should be spared ventilation if her condition means the harms she would experience cannot be justified by the expectation of benefit. Seen from the speaker's perspective, a child might represent someone whose value is so little that she does not merit ventilation. Seen from the perspective of the audience, the same child represents someone whose value is so great that she should be spared it.

Broadening what we understand by valuing a patient is one of the great contributions that consequentialist moral thinking has made to medical ethics. By introducing the concept of life 'quality', hedonistic utilitarian consequentialists in particular have drawn attention to a distinction between the value of a living person on the one hand and the value of the life that they hold on the other.[7] The term 'quality of life' is used in medicine to evaluate the benefits of interventions, many of them intangible, that are not captured by statistics about survival and, to that extent, it encompasses some of the same concepts as biographical narrative. It is intended to approximate the same broad sense of a patient's well-being and the quality of existence a patient can expect to experience if her death is postponed. Historically, 'quality of life' is an idea that has helped move medical research away from a dangerous belief that the only goal of medicine is to preserve life, or that doctors must always prolong life as long as possible, no matter what harm to the individual might be entailed by the interventions needed to achieve that prolongation. The insight that there is an important difference between being alive in the sense of enjoying existing, and being alive in the limited sense of not being dead, underpins the modern acknowledgment that compassionate medicine should not confine itself to the aim of prolonging life at all costs. Doctors are expected to consider living to be more than the mere absence of death. They must accord proper value to a living patient, and the quality of the life she is engaged in living at the time. Rather than attaching value to human life as an abstraction, clinicians should attach it to an actual individual human (they should respect the *patient's* life, rather than the patient's *life*).[8]

---

[7] Helga Kuhse, *The sanctity-of-life doctrine in medicine: a critique* (Oxford: Clarendon Press, 1987).

[8] The difference can lead to confusion in discussions between doctors and their patients. When clinicians talk about 'prognosis', they often use the same term in two quite distinct senses. One is prognosis as a measure of the probability of dying. The other is prognosis as the extent to which a patient is likely to enjoy her existence if death is delayed. Clinicians' dual understanding of prognosis is an acknowledgement that the value of an actual person, considered in her totality, is not limited to the technical value of the life that she holds, but extends to the value or quality of the sort of living she can do. To complicate things further, 'prognosis' can have a third meaning that is even more difficult to disentangle from the first; namely the probable duration of a patient's life.

10.1.1   Childness as Cognitive Impairment

So far we have said nothing about valuing cognitively impaired children that would not be equally true of cognitively impaired adults. There is nevertheless a parallel with adult-normative thinking, because a bias in favour of normal cognition represents the same arbitrary assumption that the only way to ascribe value to the way an individual experiences her life is by reference to the way a normal adult would do so.

Reasoning along adult-normative lines, there is no need to distinguish between the various ways in which a patient might fail to achieve the sort of cognition that 'counts' towards moral value. On those grounds, as we have seen, even an infant whose cognition is perfectly unimpaired still fails to make the grade as someone with full personal value. Childness itself is seen as a form of cognitive impairment. Singer, for example, does not limit his advocacy of infanticide to infants whose cognition is damaged.[9] Since he believes that all infants lack the cognitive capacities that enable adults to prefer to live, he concludes that they can—perhaps *should*—be killed if to do so would maximise preference satisfaction among adults. For society to insist that parents who do not want their infant should keep her is, Singer argues, unjust on the face of it. What makes it permissible to extinguish infants is a cognitive deficit common to all infants, damaged or otherwise. They, like animals, are 'merely conscious'.[10] Any such 'merely conscious' animal can be killed because another is sure to be born who can replace it.[11]

Although Singer is at pains to point out that it is not a child's disability that renders her apt for erasure, that argument for replaceability is of particular significance when it comes to infants who are imperfect.[12] Singer concedes that the life of

---

[9] Singer, *Practical Ethics*, p. 314.

[10] 'Many beings are sentient and capable of experiencing pleasure and pain, but they are not rational and self-conscious and, therefore, are not persons. I shall refer to these as 'merely conscious' beings. Many nonhuman animals fall into this category; so must new-born infants and some intellectually disabled humans' (Ibid., p. 85).

[11] 'When we come to animals that, as far as we can tell, lack self-awareness, the best direct reason against killing points to the loss of a pleasant or enjoyable life. Where the life taken would not, on balance, have been pleasant or enjoyable, no direct wrong is done. Even when the animal killed would have lived pleasantly, it is at least arguable that no wrong is done if the animal killed will, as a result of the killing, be replaced by another animal living an equally pleasant life. Taking this view involves holding that a wrong done to an existing being can be made up for by a benefit conferred on an as yet non-existent being. Thus, it is possible to regard merely conscious animals as interchangeable with one another in a way that beings with a sense of their own future are not'. Singer's argument for replaceability is made primarily in relation to animals. The obvious conclusion is that it is acceptable to kill animals for meat. Singer resists that conclusion, but it is because he believes that in practice animals are not happy rather than because the principle of replaceability he has set out here is not sound: 'As a piece of critical moral reasoning, this argument may be sound, but its application is limited. It cannot justify factory farming, where animals do not have pleasant lives. Nor does it normally justify the killing of wild animals' (Ibid., p. 120).

[12] 'If we favour the total view rather than the prior existence view, then we have to take account of the probability that when the death of a disabled infant will lead to the birth of another infant with better prospects of a happy life, the total amount of happiness will be greater if the disabled infant

someone with haemophilia, for example, 'can be expected to have a life worth living … His life can be expected to contain a positive balance of happiness over misery.'[13] He believes that the life of someone without haemophilia will be happier than that of a haemophiliac, so that on what he calls the 'total view', it would always be morally permissible to replace an infant who suffers from haemophilia with another infant who does not.[14]

The stigmatisation of infanticide, Singer suggests, is a noxious dogma that deprives us of a 'natural and humane' solution to the problem of unwanted or damaged babies, and is the result of wrongly ascribing inherent value to the life of such a baby just because she is human.[15] He recognises that some adults might have strong preferences against infanticide, but proposes that most of those preferences should be excluded from the preference utilitarian calculus because, although they are strongly held by large numbers of people, they are at odds with reason. Objections to a *policy* of infanticide should, he says, be set aside on logical grounds. The fact that a person can hold such a preference indicates that he himself is cognitively aware and so cannot be harmed by the policy. Objections to a specific *instance* of infanticide are irrational because, in adult-normative terms, an individual's right to life represents no more than an expression of the extent to which she prefers to continue to exist.[16] Such

---

is killed. The loss of happy life for the first infant is outweighed by the gain of a happier life for the second. Therefore, if killing the haemophiliac infant has no adverse effect on others, it would, according to the total view, be right to kill him. The total view treats infants as replaceable, in much the same way as it treats animals that are not self-aware as replaceable' (Ibid., p. 163).

[13] Ibid., p. 162.

[14] Presumably it would be not only permissible but morally required, since on the utilitarian view a moral decision that fails to maximise the desirable outcome leaves the agent as culpable as one that actively reduces it.

[15] That 'wrongly' needs to be understood in the context of Singer's wider moral theory, and particularly his commitment to animal rights. Singer is concerned that human beings have historically defined their approach to ethics largely by a commitment to considering the way they should treat other humans. On consequentialist terms, that makes no sense because the congruence between the species to which an individual belongs, and that individual's capacity to suffer, is far from perfect. While it may be generally true that human beings can suffer more than other animals because of their greater intelligence, it is not true that a human is capable of more suffering than a non-human animal simply by virtue of being human. Singer rejects as perverse the idea that we should: '… treat individuals, not in accordance with their actual qualities, but in accordance with the qualities normal for their species' (Singer, *Practical Ethics*, p. 68).

[16] 'To sum up, my argument has been that having a right to life presupposes that one is capable of desiring to continue existing as a subject of experiences and other mental states. This in turn presupposes both that one has the concept of such a continuing entity and that one believes that one is oneself such an entity. So an entity that lacks such a consciousness of itself as a continuing subject of mental states does not have a right to life'. Tooley, 'Abortion and Infanticide'. Tooley's argument here has been refuted in several different ways. John Stevens points out that a patient with a medical condition of which he has no conception might nevertheless have a right to be treated for it (J. C. Stevens, 'Must the bearer of a right have the concept of that to which he has a right?', *Ethics,* 95/1 (Oct 1984), 68–74). Christina Sommers makes the deontological argument that, in becoming parents, adults take on a moral responsibility to care for a living child (Sommers, 'Tooley's immodest proposal: Abortion and Infanticide'). Mark Tushnet and Louis Seidman sug-

objections might express the agent's spurious sense that the infant is connected to a future adult in some way that is morally relevant in the present moment, or rely on an assumption that being killed acts against the infant's interest, which Singer believes cannot be true in light of the infant's cognitive deficiencies. He concludes that the only preferences relevant to whether the infant should live or die are those of the adults on whom the impact of the infant's survival will be greatest.

The idea that childness represents a form of cognitive deficiency is not a new one. Some philosophers have equated the cognitive processes of the infant human with those of an adult human whose brain is damaged.[17] Others have compared it (to the infant's disadvantage) with the cognition of non-human animals. Bentham, for example, asserts with confidence that '... a full-grown horse or dog is beyond comparison a more rational, as well as a more conversable animal, than an infant of a day, or a week, or even a month, old'.[18] We have already seen that Tooley bases an entire thought-experiment on his assumption that the moral status of a human infant equates with that of a kitten.[19] Such assertions conveniently pathologise the state of being an infant, and so serve a polemical purpose for contemporary bioethicists who want to legitimise infanticide, but there is no scientific or philosophical basis for them. There is, in reality, little or no parallel between a human brain that is damaged, an animal brain and an infant human brain that is brand new and working perfectly. Historical medical terminology may be partly to blame here. In the past, doctors have referred to somebody whose cognition is impaired as being 'like a 5-year-old'. Of course, to anyone working with infants and children, it is clear that the term is analogical; doctors are explaining that the damage wrought on someone's brain has set a limit on how much she can develop, such that the skills that she can acquire will never be more than those of some normal 5-year-olds. They are not

---

gest that, even if the infant herself has no right to live, killing her might transgress the rights of relevant others (Tushnet and Seidman, 'A comment on Tooley's Abortion and Infanticide'). See also Davis, Nancy. 'Abortion and Infanticide (Book Review).' The Philosophical Review 94, no. 3 (1985): 436–441.

[17] For example, Engelhardt: 'When one seeks general secular grounds to justify practices through which infants, the profoundly mentally retarded, and the very senile might in general secular terms be assigned portions of the rights possessed by persons who are persons strictly, ... one is given little satisfaction' (Engelhardt, *The Foundations of Bioethics*, p. 147) and Singer: '[This] gives us a reason for preferring to use human infants–orphans perhaps–or severely retarded human beings for experiments, rather than adults, since infants and retarded humans would also have no idea of what was going to happen to them. So far as this argument is concerned nonhuman animals and infants and retarded humans are in the same category ...' (Peter Singer, *Animal liberation* (2nd edn.; London: Pimlico, 1995), p. 16). In interpreting some of these comments, it is important to note that the term 'retarded', which is offensive in the extreme in the UK, was at the time more acceptable in the USA where Engelhardt and Singer based. Furthermore, Singer is making a logical point here; he is not actually advocating that humans be used for experiments. But, while his argument is not as cold-hearted as it appears, it does recapitulate a commonly held and fundamental misbelief that normal young human cognition can be considered the same as the damaged cognition of older humans.

[18] Bentham, *An introduction to the principles of morals and legislation*, p. 311.

[19] Tooley, 'Abortion and Infanticide', p. 36.

suggesting a literal sense in which an adult brain comes to resemble the brain of a normal infant or child when it has been damaged.

That would be a somewhat bizarre claim to make. The reason a man whose brain has been damaged cannot walk is that the motor part of his brain is damaged and no longer sends signals to his legs. The reason an infant cannot walk, on the other hand, is that her perfectly functioning brain has not yet learnt to use the power that it certainly does have to control her legs. There is no connection between the two disabilities. The same is true of cognitive function; if you were to spill coffee on your much-loved and well-worn iPad, damaging its circuitry such that it no longer ran some applications, you would refer to it as an old and damaged iPad.[20] You would not equate it with the Speak & Spell you had as a child, whose functionality was limited even when it was fully operating in the way it was built to operate. Nor would you consider it to be the same as the pristine new iPad you bought to replace the damaged one, but on which you have yet to install any applications. Childness has little or nothing in common with the cognition of damaged adults or that of animals; any similarities they present to the observer are superficial and epiphenomenal.

10.1.2 Quality of Life and Its Dangers

Adult-normative thinking risks under-valuing children whose cognition is impaired for many of the same reasons that it undervalues childness itself. Because a child with a damaged brain does not appreciate or engage with the world in the same rational and autonomous way that the ideal adult would do, it is easy to assume that her enjoyment of her own existence in the moment is not as great, or as important, as that of an adult. That projection on the part of adults is difficult to disprove or to dispel, since cognitively impaired children are typically non-verbal and may be even less able than other children to communicate their subjective experiences. The inclination to value such children less highly is compounded by convenience; there is no doubt that in practice it would often make adults' lives easier if parents were permitted to instruct that their child's life be ended in the weeks following birth, where the child has complex physical and cognitive disabilities. The number of babies born prematurely or with genetic diseases is increasing, while the technology that can prevent them from dying in infancy is becoming ever more effective, so that the number of children surviving with cognitive impairment and progressive complex medical needs is growing all the time.[21] Caring for such children is emotionally exhausting and financially draining.

---

[20] Other tablet analogies are available.

[21] L. K. Fraser et al., 'Rising national prevalence of life-limiting conditions in children in England', *Pediatrics,* 129/4 (Apr 2012), e923–9, L. K. Fraser et al., *Children in Scotland requiring Palliative Care: identifying numbers and needs (The ChiSP Study)*, L. K. Fraser et al., 'Estimating the current and future prevalence of life-limiting conditions in children in England', *Palliat Med,* (Dec 15 2020), 269216320975308, L. K. Fraser and S. Jarvis, *Children with a Life-limiting or Life-threatening condition in Wales: Trends in prevalence and complexity Final report May 2023.*

One danger of the idea of evaluating life quality is the human temptation to think we know what makes someone else's life worth living or—more importantly in this context—the temptation to think we know that someone else's life is *not* worth living. In much the same way that the idea of biographical narrative broadens our understanding of the range of ways in which humans can appreciate their existence, the idea of quality of life widens our understanding of personal value beyond the value of a life to how an individual enjoys living. If, however, quality is expressed merely as a single dimension such as happiness or pleasure, the concept it represents is still implausibly narrow. It can only ever represent a fraction of the ways in which different individuals can enjoy existing. The reductive nature of some concepts of quality of life presents a particular danger to patients who are not the main decision-makers over themselves and are vulnerable to assumptions made by those around them regarding how they enjoy their own life. We have seen that Tooley and his adherents, in particular, are highly selective about the cognitive capacities that they consider can 'count' towards enjoying existence.[22] Age-neutral reasoning concludes that personal value does not represent any one specific mode in which an individual appreciates and engages with the universe, but rather the fact that an individual appreciates and engages meaningfully at all; that is, in a way that enables her to enjoy her existence in the present moment. On age-neutral terms, the fact of a doctor's obligation to consider a particular child's interests is not contingent on the precise way in which that child experiences the world. The doctor cannot therefore decide that a certain child's abilities or lack of them mean her

---

[22] 'If a being is incapable of conceiving of itself as existing over time, we need not take into account the possibility of it worrying about the prospect of its future existence being cut short. It can't worry about this, for it has no conception of its own future' (Ibid., p. 78). Critics point out that if the moral status of personhood is restricted to those who are self-aware, then any being will lose that status, not only by being unconscious as a result of illness or injury, but simply by being asleep. In his response to the Giubilini article, Catholic philosopher of law John Finnis argues that it is impossible to resist that 'repugnant or absurd conclusion' if, as Tooley and Singer insist, moral wrongness depends only on the experienced harm an action will inflict (John Finnis, 'Capacity, harm and experience in the life of persons as equals', *J Med Ethics,* 39/5 (May 2013), 281–3). Tooley anticipates such a criticism in the original exposition of his theory, though he does not provide a defence: '… an individual's right to X can be violated not only when he desires X, but also when he would desire X were it not for one of the following: (i) he is in an emotionally unbalanced state; (ii) he is temporarily unconscious; (iii) he has been conditioned to desire the absence of X' (Tooley, 'Abortion and Infanticide', p. 48). Utilitarian medical ethicist John Harris, however, refutes the criticism on the grounds that someone who is asleep has '… not necessarily lost the capacity to value life. It is a fact about human capacities and powers that it is correct to attribute them to individuals at times when they are not exercising those capacities or powers' (John Harris, *The value of life* (London: Routledge & Kegan Paul, 1985), p. 25). In an unexpected congruence with the idea of potential, Harris' argument here seems to appeal to a 'capacity or power', possession of which is a matter of fact in the present moment, even if the capacity or power is not currently being exercised. Physician Daniel Cox considers Harris' to be an inadequate response, because it relies too heavily on a distinction between an individual's being able to do something and their possessing the capacity (or potential) to be able to do it (D. R. Cox, 'The problems with utilitarian conceptions of personhood in the abortion debate', *J Med Ethics,* 37/5 (May 2011), 318–20). See also D. B. Hershenov and R. J. Hershenov, 'If Abortion, then Infanticide', *Theor Med Bioeth,* 38/5 (Oct 2017), 387–409. Hershenov argues, contra Singer, Tooley and Giubilini, that morally wrong actions can be done even to beings who are 'mindless'.

interests are not relevant, or conclude on that basis that it is permissible to withhold or withdraw treatment. Without making some personal judgement about how persons 'ought' to enjoy their lives, there is no reason to consider that the way in which a child who is cognitively impaired does so is any less valuable than the way in which any other child (or indeed adult) might do so. It would be hard to justify defining a child, still less a category of child, who should never be admitted to intensive care, because it represents a personal judgement that the enjoyment of living for children who are cognitively impaired is less important or less valuable than the enjoyment of children who are cognitively unimpaired. The statement 'we should never prolong the life of children with cognitive impairment' is, on those grounds, morally little different from 'I personally prefer children who are cognitively normal'.

10.1.3   Rationing and Cognitive Impairment

Intensivists often feel under pressure to 'ration' access to intensive care beds, on the basis that the paraphernalia needed for intensive care support represents a scarce resource for which demand exceeds availability.[23] Such pressure can contribute to a willingness to consider some children to be more valuable than others on the basis of their cognitive ability.

If we reject the idea that some ways of enjoying existence are inherently better than others, it is clear that there cannot be a simple straight-line correlation between an individual's cognitive ability and the degree to which they merit admission to intensive care. Impaired cognition is not reliably linked to impaired enjoyment of living, any more than normal cognition is a guarantee that existence will always be pleasurable.[24] In that case there is no justification for my colleague's suggestion that there should be a blanket policy of restricting cognitively impaired children's access to intensive care. Nor is it justifiable for a resource to be withheld from an actual child who is cognitively impaired in order to ensure a bed remains available to a hypothetical future child whose cognition is normal. A doctor's obligation is to concern herself with the interests of the patient in front of her and does not extend to making value judgements about what sort of living, relative to other sorts of living, succeeds or fails to justify the use of resources.

There might nevertheless be conditions under which intensivists are right to withhold or withdraw intensive care interventions from a child on the basis of cognitive impairment. One such situation is where 'triage ethics' obtains; that is, where there are two or more children who would benefit from intensive care, but only one set of equipment is available. Faced with the appalling necessity of having to withhold an intervention from a child who would benefit from it, the intensivist is right to make a judgement about which of them is likely to derive the most benefit and,

---

[23] See, for example, L. Kirby et al., 'Rationing in the Pediatric Intensive Care Unit-ethical or unethical?', *Transl Pediatr,* 10/10 (Oct 2021), 2836–44.

[24] Amy Mullin, 'Children and the Argument from 'Marginal' Cases', *Ethical Theory and Moral Practice,* 14/3 (2011), 291–305.

while cognitive ability alone should not be the only determining factor, it is a relevant consideration to the extent that it impacts on such benefit.

Triage ethics is an everyday reality for paediatricians in regions of many resource-poor countries. Elsewhere, it is not clear how often, in reality, situations occur in which triage ethics obtains. It only obtains if two or more actual and proximate individuals would both benefit from the same equipment at the same time, and only one instance of the equipment is available. Triage ethics does not obtain simply because, in the grand scheme of things, demand exceeds provision. It does not obtain if there is a vacant bed within reach of the second child, even if it would require an ambulance to get the child there. Nor does it obtain while there are intensive care beds that are occupied by children on whom ventilation is inflicting more harms than benefit, but whose parents have requested that it should continue.

On the face of it, that seems to lead to the vitalist position that as a general rule there is no child, however badly her brain is damaged, who should not be kept alive for as long as possible and by any means possible. If, as I am suggesting here, we usually refuse to consider a patient less valuable because he is cognitively impaired, surely we are committed to the idea that every life should be prolonged by intervention until the body that supports it gives out? That is only true if we confuse or conflate the two separate sorts of valuation we separated earlier. One is a judgement about how seriously the agent should take the wants, needs and desires of a patient in the first place; that is, the value of the living person. The other is a judgement about how the abilities of the specific person impact on what actions are in her interests. It is quite consistent to judge that the moral agent should concern herself with the interests of a child with cognitive impairment, and so recognise and appropriately respond to her inherent value, while at the same time acknowledging that the way in which a doctor should behave towards a child in order to serve her interests will be determined in part by her cognitive abilities. A child's abilities are material to what decisions a doctor should make, but only to the extent that they impact what is at stake.

Rationing intensive care resources on the basis of a hierarchy of value is rarely justified. Intensivists are, however, right to withhold or withdraw interventions from a child if the nature of a specific child's impairment means that child will, on balance, be harmed by the intervention. Tracheostomy is a good illustration. After some months of invasive ventilation, it is sometimes necessary to consider whether or not to make a surgical incision and insert the tube directly into the airway via the neck rather than through the mouth or nose. That can allow a child to leave the hospital and be ventilated at home, but the procedure is uncomfortable and the process of recovery and training afterwards typically takes many weeks or months, during which the child is uncomfortable and remains on the hospital ward. Since the harms are proximate, the answer to the question 'should the doctors do a tracheostomy?' will depend on whether or not the child's condition makes it likely she will survive long enough to enjoy its remoter benefits. One child might have a non-progressive brain injury, while another with precisely the same respiratory needs might have a rapidly degenerating neurological condition. Both children will experience the immediate harms of tracheostomy, but only one is likely to live long enough to experience its benefits. In the first child, tracheostomy is an act that furthers the child's interests. In the second, it is an act that will cause the child net harm. A doctor who values both children equally will accordingly respond to that value by performing a tracheostomy in one child and withholding it from the other. The difference does not, as some suggest, indicate that the doctor values the children differently.[25]

The converse might, incidentally, also be true. There are circumstances under which cognitive impairment might actually protect a child from certain harms. The unpleasantness of invasive intubation and ventilation, for example, owes at least as much to existential factors such as fear as it does to physical pain. Those existential factors are a result of processing that an anencephalic infant, to take Singer's example, cannot plausibly do in the absence of the necessary anatomical equipment. The truly anencephalic infant cannot feel his life to be in danger, or be fearful of what is happening, in the way that a normal infant can.[26] When the interests of the anencephalic infant are considered paramount in the same way as those of the normal infant, the clinician might reasonably conclude that they do not militate for or against intubation and ventilation of the anencephalic infant, because he will not experience the same harms as a normal infant might. In order to value both normal and anencephalic infants equally, the clinician might again find herself needing to make two quite different decisions.

---

[25] Peter Singer seems to believe that the only reason a doctor might withhold or withdraw an intervention that could prolong biological life is because the doctor does not value the patient highly enough to continue: 'The problem is not with the distinction that is being drawn, at least not when it is stated in terms of which means are proportionate, and which are not, to the benefit gained by extending a human life. That we should draw such a distinction is, of course, in accordance with consequentialist thinking. The point is that the way the distinction is applied is inconsistent with the idea that all human life is of equal value. For the distinction is standardly used to justify withdrawing life support from, for example, a baby with anencephaly, or from an adult with no prospect of recovering consciousness. In many of these cases, intensive medical care can prolong the life of the human organism for years, or even decades. If the patient were conscious, communicative, and capable of enjoying his or her life, we would never consider it legitimate to withdraw life support when the patient might still live for years or decades'. Peter Singer, 'Engaging with Christianity', in John Perry (ed.), *God, the good, and utilitarianism: perspectives on Peter Singer* (Cambridge: Cambridge University Press, 2014). Elsewhere, Singer makes the same claim about infants: 'The evidence [that infanticide would not disturb the entire lives of opponents of infanticide] is that infants with severe disabilities are allowed to die'. Daniel Johnson, 'Putting A Value On Human and Animal Life', http://standpointmag.co.uk/dialogue-julyaugust11-putting-a-value-on-human-life-peter-singer-nigel-biggar-euthanasia-genocide-infanticide-animal-rights--huma#comment-25682, accessed 2nd November 2015. It is not clear what Singer means, since most infant deaths in hospital could not be avoided; there is no meaningful sense in which such deaths are chosen or allowed. It is possible that Singer wrongly believes that medical interventions that might prolong life are routinely withheld from disabled infants with the primary purpose of extinguishing them rather than (as is the case) because the interventions themselves would do the infant more harm than good.

[26] It is not clear whether the truly anencephalic infant can experience pain. The part of the brain specialised for pain sensation (the thalamus) is absent in children with severe anencephaly, but some children with anencephaly nevertheless respond as though they were experiencing it. For the purposes of this discussion, I have assumed that perfect analgesia can be achieved during invasive interventions in any infant, whether anencephalic or not, so that pain is not a factor in reaching a decision regarding interests.

10.2   The Meaning of Parent, and the Role of a Doctor

Global responses to the case of Charlie Gard in the United Kingdom revealed deep fault lines in how society considers who should decide what interventions a doctor should or should not perform on a child.[27] Most commentators acknowledge that such disagreement between doctors and parents is rare. In the majority of cases where a decision needs to be made, there is no conflict. Everyone concerned with the child's interests agrees on what is best for the child and the question of whose decision it is does not arise. The decision 'makes itself' because everyone concerned with caring for the child agrees that it is the obviously correct course. Nevertheless, analysis of cases where there is conflict is important because they illustrate certain ways of thinking about a child. Generally speaking, such analyses are of three sorts. The first, played out on social media rather than representing a credible medical conversation, is a sort of conspiracy theory that suggests that doctors are in collusion with the government to save money by prematurely ending a patient's life.[28] There is no need to look at that in any detail; at best, it represents a misunderstanding and at worst deliberate misinformation. Two other ways of analysing the issue seem more plausible. One is that it hinges on a question of parental autonomy. On that view, for doctors to override parental preferences would be to fail to respect parents' right to self-rule and so would transgress one of Beauchamp and Childress' four principles. Diametrically opposed to that analysis is the idea that deciding who makes the decision is primarily a question of the responsibility of healthcare professionals to protect children from harm. On that view, the preferences of parents should simply be set aside if doctors feel the result of acting on them would probably be to cause avoidable harm to the child. On the first view, where there is conflict, it must always be the parents who decide. On the second, it must always be doctors.

Unfortunately, neither analysis takes us very far. The first represents a confused attempt to apply a traditional, adult-normative understanding of justice and respect for autonomy in which the fact of adults' moral authority to make decisions over children is often taken for granted, and the second an understanding of beneficence and non-maleficence that takes no account of the numinous and interpersonal nature of interests in children.[29]

---

[27] Gard (A Child) Re [2017] EWHC 1909 (Fam) (24 July 2017).

[28] One example among many in the Gard case is https://www.realclearhealth.com/articles/2018/05/10/british_babies_offer_cautionary_tale_on_single_payer_110786.html (accessed January 2025).

[29] Although even in principlism it is not always clearly explained. Baines, 'Medical ethics for children: applying the four principles to paediatrics'.

10.2.1   *Relevant Adults: The Meaning of Parent and the Role of a Doctor*

Adult-normative thinking can resolve conflict relatively easily by setting aside the question of the child's own interests and appealing instead to notions of ownership by adults, or adult autonomy, or by narrowing the sort of interests that the doctor needs to consider so that they encompass only what parents want for the child. Reasoning along those lines can lead to the convenient conclusion that it is morally permissible for parents to make medical decisions over their child unilaterally.

Abandoning adult-normativity complicates things. The doctor is under an obligation to act in the interests of the child, despite the fact that the nature of the child is such that it is not always possible to know what his interests are, or to disentangle them entirely from the interests of adults. Taking an age-neutral approach to the ethics of decision-making seems to put the doctor caring for a child in an impossible moral position.

Conceding that we cannot know a patient's subjective experiences entirely or with certainty, however, is not the same as saying we cannot know anything about them at all. Perhaps in the future, technology will make it possible for us to access a child's thoughts directly. For the time being, we are, to a certain extent, able to infer those subjective interests through observation, empathy and good reasoning. The infant's behaviour patterns can show pain, distress, happiness and a wide range of nuanced experiences that represent her interests. The adults who are most likely to 'get it right' (that is, to infer correctly what the child is experiencing) are those who are most familiar with the child. That is usually a child's parents, because the relationship between infant and parents is such that it is they who are the most likely to recognise a child's behaviour patterns and to interpret them correctly.

On age-neutral terms, that is what the term 'parent' stands for. It is a compassionate expert in the individual infant or child; the adult who knows better than anyone else what his subjective experiences might be, and who is the object of the infant's greatest trust. Usually, those are the adults who habitually care for the child, typically because of their biological or adoptive relationship. Since healthcare professionals have an obligation to take a child's subjective experience into account when deciding whether or not to intervene, it follows that they have an obligation to draw on the expertise that parents offer. It is clear that doctors must not make decisions over children without soliciting the observations of parents and, in most countries today, parents are recognised as expert colleagues and partners in their child's medical care whose opinions on the interests of their child are actively sought and are influential in medical decision-making.

10.2.2   Dialogue

One risk of seeking parents' expertise is that it inadvertently reinforces ideas of ownership. The authority that parents are offered over medical decisions is, or should be, a function (in the mathematical sense) of their expertise in the child's interests. It should express their special knowledge of the child in question, their ability to infer correctly the child's subjective experiences of the world and on that basis their willingness and ability to articulate what the child actually does want. It should not represent a form of tacit collusion in the idea that parents own their child. They are being consulted about a child who is 'theirs' only in the sense that they have been discharging a responsibility to care for her, and in the course of doing so have become expert in some aspects of what will benefit her most. That collegial relationship can superficially resemble a proprietary one, and it is easy for it to regress into an arrangement in which parents are accorded the authority of ownership. Instead of asking parents for their expert opinion about what would be best for the child, doctors can find themselves asking simply what the parents want. Similarly, instead of participating in collegial decision-making by helping establish what a child's interests are in discussion with the medical team, parents can find themselves expecting to give instructions to the medical team about their preferences. The effect can be that parents are given authority to influence decisions that are no longer wholly explainable or justifiable on age-neutral ethical grounds. To the extent that the authority given to parents exceeds the value of their specialist expertise, it is no longer explained by their care for or knowledge of the child and is based instead on notions of ownership.

A potential problem with the idea of parent as a compassionate expert in the child is that it is not always true. The syndrome of factitious induced illness by carers, for example, describes a well-recognised clinical situation in which a parent repeatedly brings his child to the attention of doctors because he himself achieves some gain by doing so.[30] The parent may be prepared to harm the child, often seriously, in order to support his claim that the child is unwell, and it is not uncommon for the child's death to result.[31]

That situation is unusual, and it is rare for parents consciously or deliberately to desire harm for their child. Nevertheless, the concept of trust does not offer an obvious ethical bulwark against potential abuse–deliberate or otherwise–within dependent relationships. The reality is that there are circumstances under which the

---

[30] The syndrome of FII was first characterised in children by Dr Roy Meadows in 1977. Munchausen Syndrome was already a well-recognised psychological condition in adults, in which patients would repeatedly present themselves to medical attention, often going to considerable lengths and causing themselves significant harm in the process. The syndrome was named after author Rudolf Raspe's semi-fictional fantasist, Baron Munchausen. An alternative name for FII is Munchausen Syndrome by Proxy.

[31] C. Bass and D. Glaser, 'Early recognition and management of fabricated or induced illness in children', *Lancet,* 383/9926 (Apr 19 2014), 1412–21.

interests of the child and parents are distinct and unavoidably conflict, and that opportunities abound for exerting pressure.[32] That pressure can be of all kinds: deliberate or inadvertent, well-intentioned or malign, altruistic or solipsistic, and an account of bioethics that permits delegation of medical decisions to others does not easily provide protection against it. The regrettable truth is that at the time a decision needs to be taken, especially at the end of a child's life, some parents express a preference for a course of action that is likely to inflict unjustifiable harm on a child in their care. It is not usually deliberate, but rather a consequence of the anguish they themselves are going through, which prevents them from fully assimilating the relevant facts, or leads them to interpret their own preferences as though they were synonymous with the child's interests.

An adult is not functioning as a parent when, in the midst of her grief, she says that she does not care how much her child suffers so long as she herself can postpone the pain of being finally separated from him. The nature of what we mean by 'parent' means that such a preference is not one a parent is entitled to have. In order to speak as parents, adults have an obligation to set aside their own preferences in the matter, and to represent only the interests of the child.

There is a further risk that resolving decision-making authority into two voices— that of the medically expert adult on the one hand and of the compassionate expert in the child on the other—inappropriately dichotomises the sort of expertise which only parents can bring to the discussion on the one hand, and on the other the expertise that any rational adult can offer. It is reasonable to assume as a 'rule of thumb' that doctors know more about the medical condition and its biological impact on the individual child in question, and to assume that parents know more than healthcare staff about their own child's subjective experiences. But while both of those are *generally* true, neither of them is *universally* true. It is not uncommon for parents, through long experience, to become experts in their child's condition to an extent that they know more about it than most of the healthcare team. Less intuitively, perhaps, there are also situations in which the converse is true; circumstances under which it is healthcare professionals rather than parents who are more likely to estimate a child's subjective interests accurately. That might happen, for example, when a child has been on an inpatient unit for long enough for the healthcare team, especially nurses, to have time to become familiar with the child.

The obligation to act in a child's interests means that, on age-neutral grounds, a parent is not entitled to make unilateral healthcare decisions over a child. Leaving it to doctors to make medical decisions would certainly simplify matters but, on age-neutral terms, practical convenience is not enough on its own to explain such

---

[32] Where there is a power imbalance in a relationship, there is always a risk of coercion, intentional or otherwise. Beauchamp and Childress suggest that even an adult patient's trust in a physician can militate against her capacity for self-rule. Implicit in that relationship is a power imbalance because the physician is healthy and knowledgeable, and therefore influential, while the patient is sick and lacks knowledge, and therefore vulnerable (Beauchamp and Childress, *Principles of Biomedical Ethics*, p. 100).

authority. A doctor's authority, like a parent's, is coextensive with her ability and willingness to represent the child's interests.

10.2.3   Dissensus and the Courts

On age-neutral grounds, then, neither parents nor doctors can take decisions over a child alone, because the authority of both to speak for the child is restricted to making an estimation as to what will actually help, and that requires both to know more about the child than either can muster alone. Yet the decisions still need to be taken. It follows that the only ethically correct way in which a medical decision over an infant or child can be made is in collaborative dialogue. Its purpose is to identify with as much confidence as possible what course of action is likely to offer a child the greatest excess of benefit over harm.[33] It is not for parents to give instructions to the healthcare team, or solely to set out their own preferences in the matter, or to define what the important outcomes are. Nor is it for doctors to inform parents of decisions that have already been taken, or to seek permission to withdraw harmful interventions, or to give the illusion of joint decision-making providing parents make a decision the doctors feel is 'right'. It is not even primarily to establish areas of agreement between doctor and parents, though that is often helpful. It is to establish as far as possible what is likely to be best for the child in terms that are absolute and do not depend on the personal preferences of the adults around her.

Dependence on dialogue inevitably means there must be a system for resolving dissensus when it occurs. Most commentators agree that there must be some room for parents to choose a course of action other than what is favoured by the healthcare team. But the extent to which healthcare teams should be willing to enact parents' preferences, even where they believe those preferences to be for an action that will harm the child, is contentious. Paediatric clinical ethicist Lynn Gillam describes a 'zone of parental discretion' in which there is reasonable disagreement between parent and doctor about whether an action represents harm at all.[34] Under those circumstances, she suggests, it is the preferences of parents that should prevail. Some authors go further, suggesting that there are circumstances in which harms to a child should be permitted, even if they are certain, providing they are trivial and outweighed by significant benefits to parents.[35] A challenge here is the question of treatment that is neither helping nor actively harming the child. That might include, for example, a child in whom neurological damage has progressed to a point where he is in a persistent vegetative state and is no longer able even to experience pain.

---

[33] Richard David William Hain, 'Voices of moral authority: parents, doctors and what will actually help', *Journal of Medical Ethics,* 44/7 (2018).

[34] Lynn Gillam, 'The zone of parental discretion: An ethical tool for dealing with disagreement between parents and doctors about medical treatment for a child', *Clinical Ethics,* 11/1 (2016), pp. 1–8.

[35] R. D. W. Hain, 'Parental discretion', *Arch Dis Child,* (Apr 25 2022).

The harms to the child of continuing invasive ventilation under those circumstances are relatively trivial and, on the terms proposed by Gillam, it should fall within the zone of parents' discretion. That leaves open the question of who should bear the considerable cost of continuing if that is what parents prefer. In a private healthcare system that is perhaps relatively straightforward, since the nature of the relationship between parent and healthcare provider is, to a certain extent, a contractarian one. If parents are paying for ventilation to continue, and the child is not significantly harmed by it, there seems little reason for the ethicist to quibble. But in a socialised healthcare system, the demand of justice-as-fairness is that healthcare resources are expended in the most cost-effective way possible. That cannot include continuing invasive ventilation in a patient who can no longer benefit. One solution might be a private inpatient facility that allows parents to choose to pay for futile ventilation to continue, providing it is not causing harm to their child.

If dialogue fails to achieve consensus, parents and clinicians often turn to the Court for to arbitrate. That enables their views to be heard. It forces both sides to focus on what is best for the child rather than their own preferences and ultimately resolves complex considerations into a clear plan of action that has the force of law behind it. Introducing the Courts into the system, however, brings its own problems. There is a risk that the Courts can codify ethically problematic societal assumptions about what constitutes an interest. In his book *Critically Ill Children and the Law*, legal adviser James Cameron suggests that Courts are inconsistent in the way they conceive of a child's interests, even across legislatures that share a foundation in English common law. Cameron presents evidence from his own research that Courts in Australia and New Zealand are more likely than those in the UK to discount broader aspects of the quality of a child's existence, and to privilege biological over biographical interests. He suggests that 'The lack of explanation of the interests being protected means there is a lack of transparency in the values that inform judicial decisions … further explanation of the child's relevant interests and why the state should protect these interests is required'.[36] Cameron's solution is to appeal to relevant rights that have already been agreed: the right to life, the right not to be subjected to inhuman treatment, the right to non-discrimination, the right to health, the right to lead a full and decent life for children with a disability, and the right to preserve an identity and to enjoy culture and beliefs. The effect of assessing the value of medical intervention by appeals to rights, Cameron suggests, would be to force Courts to recognise the relatively restricted role that simply prolonging technical life might have in improving the quality of someone's existence.

Although the Court considers the benefits and disbenefits to a child of each of the proposed approaches, ultimately its job is to mandate one single course of action. Since none of the courses of action can do what would be ideal in a perfect world, which would be to restore a child to health, the challenge facing the Court is to

---

[36] James Cameron, *Critically Ill Children and the Law: Medical decision-making and the best interests principle* (Abingdon: Routledge, 2024), p. 93. For a more detailed critique of Cameron's argument, see Richard Hain, 'Critically ill children and the law: medical decision-making and the best interests principle', *The New Bioethics,* (2024), 1–4.

decide what is the least non-ideal course; the single course of action that represents the child's 'best' interests. That singleness is essential for pragmatic reasons; if the practical *impasse* is to be resolved, someone has to decide on a specific course of action with a degree of authority that means the decision is binding on all parties. But an exclusive focus on best interests does not accurately reflect the medical reality, which is that in many cases more than one course of action might be expected to result in net benefit to the child. In carrying out its task of identifying and mandating the single *best* course of action, the Court might find itself having to reject a course of action that is second best, but is not unreasonable and which parents prefer.

Several commentators have suggested on that basis that instead of asking the question 'What course of action will probably result in a greater excess of good over harm that any other course of action?' the Courts should ask 'Will what parents ask probably cause more good than harm?'.[37] On the face of it, that seems an attractive idea because, instead of parents having to defend their preference, the burden of proof would be on doctors to show why that preference was unreasonable and should not be enacted.

A change in how Courts decide how much probable harm it is reasonable for parents to prefer would certainly enable parents to feel more empowered, but it too carries some risks. One is that it might perpetuate a false idea that the Court's role is to adjudicate between two sets of opinions held by adults, thus endorsing the adult-normative idea that harm and benefit to a child can be claimed by adults as matters of their personal judgement. The role of dialogue between adults, including in Court, should be to identify as far as possible something objectively true; namely, what will probably harm or benefit the child. It should not be a matter of considering the relative merits of two sets of subjective preferences held by adults.

The change would also introduce a new complication, because it leaves open the question of how much deficit in benefit is allowable before it becomes a harm. If option A carries a 99% chance of benefit with a 10% of harm, and option B carries a 90% chance of benefit with a 5% chance of harm, then both A and B are clearly reasonable. But what if parents prefer option C, which offers only a 20% chance of benefit and carries a 15% chance of harm? Option C, like options A and B, offers an excess of benefit over harm and so would not technically cross the harm threshold. But choosing C means the child misses out on a significant amount of benefit and is exposed to a significant amount of harm, relative to A or B. Even though C represents a course of action that would not actively harm the child, a preference for C would not be a reasonable one for parents to hold because the effect of their choice is more than just to institute C; it also denies the chance of A or B. That denial

---

[37] For a thoughtful critique of the harm threshold test, see D. Wilkinson, 'In defense of a conditional harm threshold test for paediatric decision-making.', *Parental Rights, Best Interests and Significant Harms: Medical decision-making on behalf of children post Great Ormond St vs Yates* (Oxford: Hart Publishing, 2019). Wilkinson proposes a compromise in which the willingness of a health provider to offer further treatment is taken as evidence that parents' preference for it is reasonable, even in the face of a Court's decision that it is not in a child's 'best' interests.

represents a significant harm to the child, which would be permitted by a move away from a best interests test.

The Court process, as it currently stands, is effective, but often cruel. It is cruel to parents, who can feel humiliated by the process, and to the healthcare team who are prevented by confidentiality laws from defending themselves in the public space against a charge of callous authoritarianism. Most worrying of all, from an age-neutral ethical perspective, the Court process is cruel to the child. Preparation can take many weeks or months, during which the interventions in contention are usually expected to continue, even though most will eventually be deemed by the Courts to have been the cause of more harm than could be justified by their benefit. That means that the child has had to endure several weeks of suffering that were potentially avoidable. That is something that any adult who cares for a child should agree is unacceptable.

One solution would be to introduce a process of scrutiny by a quasi-legal national 'child's interests panel' to which referrals could be made instead of the Courts. Such a panel could comprise independent doctors, lawyers, philosophers and lay representatives, whose task would be to consider what course of action would be in a child's interests, considered broadly and along the age-neutral lines we have already considered. The panel would have delegated authority from the Court, and its decisions would have to be legally binding on both parties.

10.3 Summary

There are many different ways in which an individual can appreciate and engage with the universe in order to enjoy her existence. Just as the fact that an individual exhibits only the characteristics of childness is not a reason to permit others to kill him, so the fact that an individual is cognitively impaired cannot of itself be taken as evidence that she is unable to enjoy her existence. An age-neutral argument makes the claim that the range of ways in which individual humans can enjoy their existence is much wider than many theories are willing to acknowledge. There can be an assumption that a child who cannot speak or walk cannot be experiencing their life in a way that can meaningfully be described as having quality. To those who know such children, however, their joy in relationship and existence is often obvious. If we consider broadly enough what we mean by 'biographical narrative', it becomes clear that even children with quite severe cognitive impairment are capable of doing it. It is not ethically permissible for a moral agent to be more concerned about the interests of a child whose cognitive abilities are normal than with those whose cognitive abilities are impaired, and to extinguish such a person would be to deprive someone who is already a person of the opportunity to experience her existence in the present moment.

Expressing the value of a life solely in terms of a preference to live disconnects ethics from reality. It implies that the only thing that makes an individual's life worth living is knowing that she will continue to exist in the future. That would discount altogether the moral value of capacities that enable someone to be happy, or to suffer, or simply to appreciate existing in the present moment. It is inconceivable that an individual's only morally relevant characteristic is a capacity to have preferences. Nor is the connection between well-being and preference satisfaction straightforward in the way Singer's preference utilitarianism demands. Sometimes we fail to flourish despite the fact that our rationally reached preferences were perfectly satisfied. Sometimes we flourish because of something that we did not prefer, but which happened anyway.

A commitment to valuing all patients equally does not entail a commitment to vitalism, because there is a distinction between the value of a living individual and the value of the biological life that they hold. A patient does not become unimportant to the doctor just because her life has no quality. But recognising her importance or value does not commit the doctor to introducing any and every intervention that might prolong biological life. There might well be some circumstances under which the correct and compassionate response to her importance might be for a doctor to decide not to intervene or to stop intervening; not because the doctor fails to value the patient adequately, but because the intervention represents a net harm.

Parents do not own their child, nor is there anything inherent in their biological relationship with the child that gives their voice special authority. On age-neutral terms, the authority of adults to make decisions about a child comes from two sources, and only two: the first, which parents share with any rational adult in possession of the facts, is in the extent to which they understand and are willing to articulate a child's objective interests. The second, which on age-neutral terms essentially defines what is meant by 'parent', is in the extent to which they accurately estimate a child's subjective interests. The unique authority possessed by parents is that they are usually the ones who can speak in the voice of the compassionate expert in the child. They are, in effect, world experts in their own child. On age-neutral terms, the authority of an adult to make medical decisions over a child flows from the dependence that is characteristic of childness and is co-extensive with that adult's ability and willingness to estimate correctly what action would further the child's interests.

The range of knowledge needed to make ethically defensible decisions is so wide that it would usually be impossible for a single adult. Any rational adult can, in principle, make a reasonable estimation of a child's objective interests, because these are matters of observation that do not depend on the child's own experience of the world. In a situation where a medical decision needs to be made, doctors are typically the adults who know the child's objective interests most accurately. Only adults who know a child very well indeed, on the other hand, are in a position to estimate those interests that flow from a child's subjective experiences. The purpose of dialogue between parents and healthcare professionals is to bring together estimates of a child's objective interests (usually, but not always, the expertise of healthcare professionals) and expertise regarding her subjective interests (usually, but not always, the expertise of biological parents).

When making decisions about medical interventions, the doctor has a duty to solicit the views of the child's parents, even where they are not speaking with a parental voice (that is, they are not speaking with a voice that estimates interests that arise from the child's own subjective experiences). The doctors must then evaluate parents' preferences appropriately so that, while the interests of the infant or child are paramount, the interests of parents are also given appropriate weight. On age-neutral grounds, the interests of parents must usually be suborned to the interests of the child where the two are in conflict. Most of the time, however, an infant's parents want the best for their infant, so that the interests of parents and infant are aligned, so that acting in the interests of one simultaneously enables the moral agent to act in the interests of both. It might be reasonable for parents to choose to continue interventions that no longer hold out any realistic chance of benefit to a child (providing they do not inflict significant harm), but in a socialised healthcare system that should be at parents' own expense.

The dependence on dialogue makes occasional dissensus inevitable and at the moment the only system for resolving it is often the Court. While that has many benefits, the process of preparing for Court is long, and too often delays the healthcare team from taking an action which is ultimately recognised to be the morally correct one. Cognitive impairment does not attenuate a child's capacity to suffer, and a system that allows a child to continue to endure unnecessary suffering at the hands of adults should be unacceptable. A solution is the idea of children's interest panels.

Bibliography

Baines P. Medical ethics for children: applying the four principles to paediatrics. J Med Ethics. 2008;34(3):141–5.

Bass C, Glaser D. Early recognition and management of fabricated or induced illness in children. Lancet. 2014;383(9926):1412–21.

Beauchamp T, Childress J. Principles of biomedical ethics. 6th ed. New York: Oxford University Press; 2009.

Bentham J. An introduction to the principles of morals and legislation, Principles of morals and legislation. Oxford: Clarendon Press; 1879.

Cameron J. Critically ill children and the law: medical decision-making and the best interests principle. Abingdon: Routledge; 2024.

Cox DR. The problems with utilitarian conceptions of personhood in the abortion debate. J Med Ethics. 2011;37(5):318–20.

Dening G. Giving the past its dignity. In: Malpas J, Lickiss N, editors. Perspectives on human dignity: a conversation. 1st ed. Dordrecht: Springer; 2007.

Engelhardt HT. The foundations of bioethics. New York: Oxford University Press; 1996.

Finnis J. Capacity, harm and experience in the life of persons as equals. J Med Ethics. 2013;39(5):281–3.

Francis R. Report of the Mid Staffordshire NHS Foundation Trust public inquiry. London: Stationery Office; 2013.

Fraser LK, Jarvis S. Children with a life-limiting or life-threatening condition in Wales: trends in prevalence and complexity. Final report May 2023. York: University of York; 2023.

Fraser LK, et al. Rising national prevalence of life-limiting conditions in children in England. Pediatrics. 2012;129(4):e923–9.

Fraser LK, et al. Children in Scotland requiring Palliative Care: identifying numbers and needs (The ChiSP Study). University of York Social Policy Research Unit; 2015.

Fraser LK, et al. Estimating the current and future prevalence of life-limiting conditions in children in England. Palliat Med. 2020;35:2692163209753308.

Gillam L. The zone of parental discretion: an ethical tool for dealing with disagreement between parents and doctors about medical treatment for a child. Clin Ethics. 2016;11(1):1–8.

Hain RDW. Voices of moral authority: parents, doctors and what will actually help. J Med Ethics. 2018;44(7):458.

Hain RDW. Parental discretion. Arch Dis Child. 2022;107:853.

Hain R. Critically ill children and the law: medical decision-making and the best interests principle. New Bioeth. 2024;31:67–71.

Hare RM. Freedom and reason. Oxford: Oxford University Press; 1965.

Harris J. The value of life. London: Routledge & Kegan Paul; 1985.

Hershenov DB, Hershenov RJ. If abortion, then infanticide. Theor Med Bioeth. 2017;38(5):387–409.

Johnson D. Putting a value on human and animal life. 2015. http://standpointmag.co.uk/dialogue-julyaugust11-putting-a-value-on-human-life-peter-singer-nigel-biggar-euthanasia-genocide-infanticide-animal-rights-huma#comment-25682. Accessed 2nd November.

Jones DG. The dead body as an object of investigation. In: Fitzgerald JJ, Moyse AJ, editors. Treating the body in medicine and religion: Jewish, Christian, and Islamic perspectives. 1st ed. London: Routledge; 2018.

Kirby L, et al. Rationing in the Pediatric Intensive Care Unit-ethical or unethical? Transl Pediatr. 2021;10(10):2836–44.

Kuhse H. The sanctity-of-life doctrine in medicine: a critique. Oxford: Clarendon Press; 1987.

McGee A, Gardiner D. Differences in the definition of brain death and their legal impact on intensive care practice. Anaesthesia. 2019;74(5):569–72.

Neuberger BJ, Guthrie LG, Aaronovitch D, Hameed K, Bonser T, Professor Lord Harries of Pentregarth, Charlesworth-Smith D, Professor Jackson E (2013), 'More care, less pathway: a review of the Liverpool Care Pathway', Independent Review of the Liverpool Care Pathway (Crown copyright).

Pigliucci M. RS97 – Peter Singer on being a utilitarian in the real world. 2019. http://rationallyspeakingpodcast.org/show/rs97-peter-singer-on-being-a-utilitarian-in-the-real-world.html. Accessed 21 January.

Plunkett A, Parslow RC. Is it taking longer to die in paediatric intensive care in England and Wales? Arch Dis Child. 2016;101(9):798.

Rennick JE, Childerhose JE. Redefining success in the PICU: new patient populations shift targets of care. Pediatrics. 2015;135(2):e289–91.

Singer P. Animal liberation. 2nd ed. London: Pimlico; 1995.

Singer P. Practical ethics. New York: Cambridge University Press; 2011.

Singer P. Engaging with Christianity. In: Perry J, editor. God, the good, and utilitarianism: perspectives on Peter Singer. Cambridge: Cambridge University Press; 2014.

Sommers CH. Tooley's immodest proposal: abortion and infanticide. Hast Cent Rep. 1985;15(3):39–42.

Stevens JC. Must the bearer of a right have the concept of that to which he has a right? Ethics. 1984;95(1):68–74.

Tooley M. Abortion and infanticide. Philos Public Aff. 1972;2(1):37–65.

Tushnet M, Seidman LM. A comment on Tooley's abortion and infanticide. Ethics. 1986;96(2):350–5.

Wilkinson D. In defense of a conditional harm threshold test for paediatric decision-making. In: Parental rights, best interests and significant harms: medical decision-making on behalf of children post Great Ormond St vs Yates. Oxford: Hart Publishing; 2019.

Chapter 11
Closing Comments

While a trainee in adult palliative medicine in North America, I was once asked to review Mathieu, an elderly gentleman on the oncology ward who had advanced lung cancer. Secondary deposits of his cancer had spread to his brain, robbing him of the ability to remember further than 5 min in the past. His life had become a sort of archipelago in time; a series of tiny islands through which the passage of hours and days gently but relentlessly propelled him, each one his entire world while he was on it.

Mathieu's daughter was his main carer and had asked for him to be moved to a local hospice for these last few weeks of his life. My task was to review him and start making appropriate arrangements for the transfer. Within a few minutes of my meeting him, however, Mathieu made it clear to me that he wanted to be cared for at home. He told me tearfully that he desperately wanted to be in his own house, and that his last few weeks would be unbearable if he spent them anywhere else. I left feeling profoundly uncomfortable. There was no practical reason why Mathieu should not go home; he had been cared for there for some time before his admission and the support was already in place. He could certainly be managed safely and effectively in the location of his choice. But his daughter had made her own preferences very clear. She wanted him admitted to the hospice; for her, no other option was acceptable. Over the next few days, my discomfort grew. Despite his damaged memory, Mathieu was absolutely consistent. Each time I saw him, he expressed the same passionate preference to go home and not into a hospice. I decided to arrange to meet the resident doctor on the oncology team to discuss the ethical quandary into which Mathieu had placed us.

My colleague professed herself puzzled by my dilemma. Surely there was no quandary here. There was, after all, no doubt that Mathieu lacked competence or capacity in any legal sense, nor was there any doubt that his daughter and the oncology team had the legal power and authority to admit him to a hospice. The answer was so clear that, in the view of my colleague, my reservations were simply vexatious obstacles to proceeding with what was obviously the right course of action. I

© The Author(s), under exclusive license to Springer Nature
Switzerland AG 2026
R. Hain, *Childness and the Myth of the Unfinished Human*,
https://doi.org/10.1007/978-3-032-12111-0_11

explained that although Mathieu lacked capacity, he *was* capable of being made happy by something that we were in a position to provide, and were choosing to deny him. As I saw it, I concluded, the problem with what was being proposed was not a matter of the law, but rather of ethics. At this, she lost all patience with me. Gathering up the patient's notes, she swept off to arrange a formal capacity assessment for Mathieu, pausing only to sneer over her shoulder, 'Don't talk to *me* about ethics. I have ethics to Master's level!'

I have had many similar conversations over the years. Doctors (with or without Master's degrees in ethics) are, on the whole, doers, not thinkers. Typically, we possess considerable faculty for rapidly analysing complex situations, and are good at making a judgement about what would be the best outcome for a patient, and making decisions whose objective is to make that outcome as likely as possible. But doctors are not (again, on the whole) deep or careful thinkers. Things move so fast too in clinical medicine that there is rarely time for much in the way of sophisticated ratiocination. In medicine, to 'demonstrate' something is usually considered synonymous with showing it empirically rather than, as in the humanities, being able to set out a sound chain of reasoning. In any case, generally speaking, the ethical decisions that we have to make in our day-to-day practice are pragmatic ones that make relatively few metaphysical demands. There are, of course, doctors who are also card-carrying philosophers or moral theologians, but they remain rare.

If those with medical training sometimes fall short as philosophers, perhaps there is an even greater risk that philosophers might fall short when it comes to a knowledge of medicine. Medicine is not a subject one can convincingly 'pick up' in the course of preparing a treatise on medical ethics, or considering how best to expound a new bioethical theory. Since the middle of the twentieth century, it has nevertheless often been moral philosophers, rather than physicians, who have influenced the way we think ethically about how medicine should be practised.

Nowhere is that more obvious than in medical ethics in children. While doctors or nurses are expected to undergo years of training before working with children, there is no parallel requirement in moral philosophy; no qualification to be, as it were, a paediatric bioethicist. A moral philosopher or theologian who wishes to publish theories about the inherent value of infants and children is under no professional obligation to learn anything about them, or about normal human neurodevelopment. But that sort of knowledge matters, especially to theories that seek to express individual value in terms of cognitive abilities. Without it, the degree of confidence with which accounts of the value of 'childness' in bioethical theories are sometimes expressed is not entirely justified. All too often, bioethics in infants and children has provided an example of what Peter Singer terms 'reaching conclusions from the armchair on a topic that demands investigation in the real world'.[1] When it comes to ensuring debate in medical ethics is well-informed from both sources, it cannot be the exclusive preserve of the abstract philosopher any more than of the practical clinician. Each needs to be properly informed by the other. It is just as

---

[1] Singer, *Practical Ethics*, p. 228.

important that moral philosophy and theology are disciplined by an understanding of medical practice as it is for medical practice to be disciplined by an understanding of ethics. That is perhaps especially important in the face of the growing influence of consequentialism in medical ethics. In the past, philosophers tended to appeal to metaphysics in defence of their hypotheses, while scientists preferred to invoke empirical evidence. One attraction of a consequentialist approach to bioethics has been that it makes it easy to set metaphysics aside, thus putting the ethics that underpins medicine on the same empirical footing as the science. Medical science has yet, perhaps, to make a reciprocal concession to the value of metaphysics.

There are omissions from this book that some readers might find surprising. One is that I have not addressed the issue of children's rights. A medical student on a paediatric placement once challenged me to declare myself a 'rights enthusiast' or a 'rights sceptic'. I found the question more difficult to answer than she anticipated. As a paediatrician, of course, I applaud the idea of children's rights. They are levers to influence legislation so that children are treated with the respect and compassion they deserve. They are assertions that we should waste no more time on academic moral debate; that further philosophical discussion would be otiose and counterproductive. A rights claim is a statement that the results of moral reasoning are in, and we know what is right when it comes to moral actions regarding children.

But, while the paediatrician in me is a rights enthusiast, the ethicist in me is a sceptic for precisely the same reasons. The idea of rights is predicated on the notion that the moral agent should treat an individual in a certain way because that individual belongs to a certain category. The rights of a British citizen to be treated in certain ways depend on her being British, for example, and are not changed by whether or not a specific British citizen can benefit from being treated in those ways. Claiming a right represents a sort of leapfrogging or bypassing of moral reasoning. It seeks to jump directly from the situation in which an individual finds herself to an unambiguous decision about what actions should be taken, without any of the intervening logical thought. There is a sense in which claims of rights are antithetical to careful moral reasoning rather than adjuncts to it.

Unwisely, I once voiced my philosophical misgivings to a passionate rights enthusiast. She rounded on me furiously and it became clear that, as far as she is concerned, expressing any kind of scepticism about rights is tantamount to being an apologist for the exploitation of children. At the time I was somewhat taken aback by the onslaught. Reflecting on it afterwards, I wondered if two somewhat separate ideas had become confused. The reservations I had expressed were in respect of the way in which specific rights have been claimed. While sometimes that has been on the basis of clear empirical evidence, or on sound moral reasoning from axioms about the child's nature, quite often adults have sought to claim rights for children simply because they represent an expression of how, in their own opinion, children should be treated. The moral authority of that second sort of rights claim must be considered more questionable than that of the first, and (*contra* my colleague) it seems to me legitimate to hold to rational account any or all of the specific rights that are claimed for children, particularly if they are to have legal force.

Where my colleague and I would emphatically agree, however, is that the nature of children is such that they can have rights, and that those rights can be held against adults—even their parents. That is a radical and foundational claim about the value of an individual child. But it is also a radical and foundational claim about the value of *being* a child; of the distinctive value of a child's nature that needs no reference to the value of being an adult. It is an assertion that to exist as a child is just as valuable a way of being a person (for the purposes of this discussion, a *human* person) as existing as an adult. So, while I have not attempted a critique of rights as such, the argument I have set out in this book should certainly be taken as an endorsement of the idea that children do have rights, and that those rights arise from their nature as children, independently of any reference to, or relationship with, the adults around them.

Another topic I have chosen not to address in this book is abortion. That is not only because it is an incendiary topic on which everything that can be said has already been said. Nor is it because my sex, gender and circumstances mean the question is unlikely to be personally relevant. It is because I do not think what I have to say in this book contributes materially to the debate. That might seem surprising, given that my main thesis is that even newborn infants appreciate and engage with the world in a way that enables them to experience and enjoy a distinctively human existence. Surely, if I am suggesting that newborn babies are meaningfully aware, I must extend the same conclusion to fetuses, at least in the later stages of gestation?

We do not know if I would be correct in drawing such a conclusion, of course. But even we did know—if a device were available that enabled us to know exactly what a fetus was thinking—I do not think it would change the abortion argument significantly. Those who suggest abortion should always be illegal already believe that the fetus has the same moral status as an adult. Those who believe there should be no restriction on abortion see it exclusively as a question of a woman's rights over her own body; that, too, would not be changed by anything we might discover about the fetus. And most women who undergo abortion are not doing it because they feel there is no moral question (in my experience, most are only too aware of it), but because their circumstances at the time mean they feel there is no choice. Knowing how a fetus experiences existence would not change that either. Like everyone else, I have my own views on abortion, but this book was not the place to expound or explore them.

Reading an early draft of the manuscript, a colleague told me that there were times when the thought that passed through his head was 'Wow—Richard really hates consequentialism!' That would not be true; at least, it would not be wholly true. Consequentialism certainly comes in for considerable criticism in several chapters in this book, but that is because, alongside deontology and virtue ethics, it represents one of the three major philosophical approaches that have most importantly informed the 'four principles' structure, which continues to dominate medical ethics thinking. Consequentialism has often seemed keen to usurp Principlism; to unseat it as the accepted way for doctors to analyse and consider medical ethical quandaries, and to place on the throne instead a straightforward pragmatic calculus of benefits and harms. Despite the fact that some key consequentialist ideas are central to Principlism, many consequentialist philosophers have even chosen to define their position in opposition to it, and much of the debate that has characterised medical ethics in the last 50 years has in effect been a dialogue between Principlism and consequentialism. In considering how medical ethics should deal with infants and children, it seems reasonable to offer a critique of both protagonists.

Among careful and compassionate thinkers, there are both adherents to, and fierce opponents of, consequentialism as a general theory and, even if I were equipped to do so, it would have been outside the scope of this book to essay a defence of either position. It does seem to me, however, that consequentialist moral thinking in medical ethics potentially presents a special danger to infants and children. 'Consequentialism' encompasses many different theories that are distinguished from one another by what they assert as the desirable outcome of moral action.

The special danger that consequentialism presents to infants and children is that the objectives of some consequentialist theories, especially utilitarian ones, are easier to achieve in adults than they are in children. Any kind of moral theory whose objective is inevitably made easier for the agent to achieve by the beneficiary's being an adult will have no choice but to set the value of infants and children at less than that of an adult. That category of theories largely excludes deontology and virtue ethics theories, because their accounts of personal value do not depend on what the beneficiary of moral action is like. But it certainly includes some consequentialist theories; namely, those which assert a desirable outcome that is made more accessible by capacities in the beneficiary that are characteristically adult. That might include, for example, possession of a logical faculty, or the capacity to make decisions autonomously, or to make preferences.

Before leaving the subject of consequentialism, it is worth making a distinction between a theory that can correctly explain moral personal value when it is present, and one that can conclude correctly that there is no such value. A perfect theory, of course, would achieve both. And perhaps there is, or will one day be, a consequentialist theory that does so. In the meantime, while it would be hard to disagree with most consequentialist theories when they ascribe value, they tend to be less convincing when they deny it. It is one thing to observe that a certain object is valuable because it is a jewel that is hard, clear and highly refractive to light. It is another to extrapolate from that to the conclusion that a second object is not valuable because instead it is a metal that is soft, yellow and opaque, or exists only as encrypted ones and zeroes on a computer hard drive. It is one thing to observe that a person is valuable because he is autonomous; it is another to extrapolate from that to the conclusion that a second person is not valuable because he is dependent.

The scepticism that my colleague identified is an expression of my concern about the ability of some of the specific consequentialist theories that currently influence medical ethics to evaluate infants and children correctly. Consequentialism is a highly vocal protagonist in modern bioethical conversation, and one important aim of this book is to hold it to account for some of the claims that have been made in its name about the value of infants and children. In doing so, I have often had to think and write like a consequentialist and at times to defend consequentialist logic; it seems obvious that such logic has an important place in medical ethics. I would not, however, consider myself a consequentialist. I agree with Beauchamp and Childress that medical ethics needs to turn to a wider range of moral theories; theories that can account for value in ways that strictly consequentialist theories do not. Most consequentialist theories in medical ethics at the moment start with an attempt to simplify the way in which persons experience their existence and to express it in terms of a single idea, such as happiness, or autonomy, or preference satisfaction. But the defining feature of humans' experience of existence is not simplicity but complexity. It seems hypothetically possible that a certain sort of 'eudaimonic consequentialism' could encompass the countless different ways in which humans can flourish, which would ensure that bioethics minimises the risk of wrongly ascribing a zero value to the life or existence of some patients. In practice, I think it would be hard to find a consequentialist theory whose desirable outcome was so capacious, and yet so universally applicable, that it could describe the valuable and the valueless with equal accuracy, or be able to distinguish between them with kind of reliability demanded by a moral endeavour such as medical ethics whose end result can determine someone's life or death. As must have become clear in this book, it seems to me that a form of consequentialism based on the idea of biographical narrative comes closer than most.

American humourist Franklin Jones once remarked that: 'Children are unpredictable. You never know what inconsistency they're going to catch you in next'. I have argued that modern bioethics is implicitly biased in favour of adult ways of thinking and being. I have traced this bias to philosophical traditions that equate moral worth with certain forms of cognitive function but not others, and so marginalise those whose experiences differ from the adult norm. It is a way of thinking that inevitably leads to the undervaluation of children—especially infants—in moral reasoning and medical practice and as a result it is profoundly dangerous. Medical ethics must abandon that adult-normative paradigm and embrace instead an age-neutral moral anthropology that is grounded not only in compassion but in evidence, and the recognition that all human beings—regardless of the precise way in which they appreciate and enjoy their own existence—possess inherent moral worth.

Bibliography

Agar N. How to insure against utilitarian overconfidence. Monash Bioeth Rev. 2014;32(3–4):162–71.

Akbari H, et al. Towards reconstructing intelligible speech from the human auditory cortex. Sci Rep. 2019;9(1):874.

Anand KJ, Carr DB. The neuroanatomy neurophysiology and neurochemistry of pain stress and analgesia in newborns and children. Pediatr Clin North Am. 1989;36(4):797–822.

Anand KJ, Hickey PR. Pain and its effects on the human neonate and fetus. N Engl J Med. 1987;317(21):1321–9.

Anderson JR. The development of self-recognition: a review. Dev Psychobiol. 1984;17(1):35–49.

Archard D. John Locke's children. In: Turner SM, Matthews GB, editors. The philosopher's child: critical perspectives in the Western tradition. Rochester/Woodbridge: University of Rochester Press; 1998.

Archard D. Children. In: LaFollette H, editor. The Oxford handbook of practical ethics. Oxford: Oxford University Press; 2005.

Aristotle. Politics, Loeb classical library; trans. Rackham H. Cambridge, MA: Harvard University Press; 1932.

Aristotle. Nicomachean ethics, Cambridge texts in the history of philosophy; trans. Crisp R. Cambridge: Cambridge University Press; 2000.

Aristotle. On the generation of animals. c 350 BC.

Armour JA. The little brain on the heart. Cleve Clin J Med. 2007;74(Suppl_1):S48.

Baines P. Medical ethics for children: applying the four principles to paediatrics. J Med Ethics. 2008;34(3):141–5.

Bass C, Glaser D. Early recognition and management of fabricated or induced illness in children. Lancet. 2014;383(9926):1412–21.

Baumrind D. Parental discipline and social competence in children. Youth Soc. 1978;9:238–76.

Beauchamp TL. Principlism and its alleged competitors. Kennedy Inst Ethics J. 1995;5(3):181–98.

Beauchamp T, Childress J. Principles of biomedical ethics. 6th ed. New York: Oxford University Press; 2009.

Bentham J. An introduction to the principles of morals and legislation, Principles of morals and legislation. Oxford: Clarendon Press; 1879.

Berg JW. The legal requirements for disclosure and consent: history and current status. In: Berg JW, Appelbaum PS, editors. Informed consent: legal theory and clinical practice. 2nd ed. Oxford/New York: Oxford University Press; 2001. p. 41–74.

Berlin I. Two concepts of liberty: an inaugural lecture delivered before the University of Oxford on 31 October 1958. Oxford: Clarendon Press; 1958.

Biggar N. Aiming to kill: the ethics of suicide and euthanasia. Pilgrim Press; 2004.

Birchley G. Charlie Gard and the weight of parental rights to seek experimental treatment. J Med Ethics. 2018;44(7):448–52.

Brahams D, Brahams M. The Arthur case: a proposal for legislation. J Med Ethics. 1983;9(1):12–5.

Buolamwini J, Gebru T. Gender shades: intersectional accuracy disparities in commercial gender classification. Proc Mach Learn Res. 2018;81:1–15.

Cameron J. Critically ill children and the law: medical decision-making and the best interests principle. Abingdon: Routledge; 2024.

Camosy C. Too expensive to treat?: finitude, tragedy, and the neonatal ICU. W.B. Eerdmans Publishing Company; 2010.

Camosy C. Engaging with Peter Singer. In: Perry J, editor. God, the good, and utilitarianism: perspectives on Peter Singer. Cambridge: Cambridge University Press; 2014.

Celano A. Medieval theories of practical reason: the thomistic doctrine of practical reason. Stanford Encyclopedia of Philosophy; 2017. https://plato.stanford.edu/entries/practical-reason-med/. Accessed 1st March.

Charlton R, editor. Compassion. London: Royal College of General Practitioners; 2015.

Childress JF. Protestant perspectives on informed consent (particularly in research involving human participants). Fordham Urban Law J. 2002;30(1 art 11):187–205.

Clark SRL. The political animal: biology, ethics, and politics. London/New York: Routledge; 2001.

Coady CA. The common premise for uncommon conclusions. J Med Ethics. 2013;39(5):284–8.

Council of Europe. Convention for the protection of human rights and dignity of the human being with regard to the application of biology and medicine: convention on human rights and biomedicine, Oviedo, 4.IV.1997. Strasbourg: Council of Europe; 1997.

Cox DR. The problems with utilitarian conceptions of personhood in the abortion debate. J Med Ethics. 2011;37(5):318–20.

Darwin C. The descent of man part III (eds. Desmond AJ, Moore J). London: Penguin Classics; 2017.

Dawkins R. The selfish gene. Oxford/New York: Oxford University Press; 2006.

Dening G. Giving the past its dignity. In: Malpas J, Lickiss N, editors. Perspectives on human dignity: a conversation. 1st ed. Dordrecht: Springer; 2007.

Dennett DC. Brainstorms: philosophical essays on mind and psychology, Penguin science. London: Penguin; 1997.

Department of Health. Mental Capacity Act (2005), c.9. London: HMSO; 2008.

Droit-Volet S. Time perception in children: a neurodevelopmental approach. Neuropsychologia. 2013;51(2):220–34.

Echteld MA, et al. Quality of life change and response shift in patients admitted to palliative care units: a pilot study. Palliat Med. 2005;19(5):381–8.

Echteld MA, et al. Changes in and correlates of individual quality of life in advanced cancer patients admitted to an academic unit for palliative care. Palliat Med. 2007;21(3):199–205.

Efferson C, Lalive R, Fehr E. The coevolution of cultural groups and ingroup favoritism. Science. 2008;321(5897):1844–9.

Engelhardt HT. The foundations of bioethics. New York: Oxford University Press; 1996.

Farah MJ, Heberlein AS. Personhood and neuroscience: naturalizing or nihilating? Am J Bioeth. 2007;7(1):37–48.

Filmer R. Patriarcha and other political works. 1st ed. Oxfordshire: Routledge; 2017.

Finnis J. Capacity, harm and experience in the life of persons as equals. J Med Ethics. 2013;39(5):281–3.

Fjellstrom R. Is Singer's ethics speciesist? Environ Values. 2003;12(1):91–106.

Fletcher JF. Humanhood: essays in biomedical ethics. Prometheus Books; 1979.

Fonagy P, Gergely G, Target M. The parent-infant dyad and the construction of the subjective self. J Child Psychol Psychiatry. 2007;48(3–4):288–328.

Francis R. Report of the Mid Staffordshire NHS Foundation Trust public inquiry. London: Stationery Office; 2013.

Frankfurt HG. Freedom of the will and the concept of a person. In: Lizza JP, editor. Defining the beginning and end of life: readings on personal identity and bioethics. Baltimore: Johns Hopkins University Press; 2009.

Fraser LK, Jarvis S. Children with a life-limiting or life-threatening condition in Wales: trends in prevalence and complexity. Final report May 2023. York: University of York; 2023.

Fraser LK, et al. Rising national prevalence of life-limiting conditions in children in England. Pediatrics. 2012;129(4):e923–9.

Fraser LK, et al. Children in Scotland requiring Palliative Care: identifying numbers and needs (The ChiSP Study). University of York Social Policy Research Unit; 2015.

Fraser LK, et al. Estimating the current and future prevalence of life-limiting conditions in children in England. Palliat Med. 2020;35:269216320975308.

Friedman SH, Cavney J, Resnick PJ. Mothers who kill: evolutionary underpinnings and infanticide law. Behav Sci Law. 2012;30(5):585–97.

Gallup GG Jr. Chimpanzees: self-recognition. Science. 1970;167(3914):86–7.

General Medical Council. Good medical practice. London: General Medical Council; 2023.

Gillam L. The zone of parental discretion: an ethical tool for dealing with disagreement between parents and doctors about medical treatment for a child. Clin Ethics. 2016;11(1):1–8.

Gillon R. Medical ethics: four principles plus attention to scope. Br Med J. 1994;309:184–8.

Gillon R. Ethics needs principles—four can encompass the rest—and respect for autonomy should be "first among equals". J Med Ethics. 2003;29(5):307–12.

Giubilini A, Minerva F. After-birth abortion: why should the baby live? J Med Ethics. 2013;39(5):261–3.

Goksan S, et al. fMRI reveals neural activity overlap between adult and infant pain. elife. 2015;4:e06356.

Gopnik A. Why babies are more conscious than we are. Behav Brain Sci. 2007;30(5–6):503–4.

Gopnik A. The philosophical baby: what children's minds tell us about truth love & the meaning of life. London: Bodley Head; 2009.

Green RM. Stem cell research: a target article collection part III – determining moral status. Am J Bioeth. 2002;2(1):20.

Green B. Use of the Hippocratic or other professional oaths in UK medical schools in 2017: practice, perception of benefit and principlism. BMC Res Notes. 2017;10(1):777.

Greenberg DM, et al. Testing the Empathizing-Systemizing theory of sex differences and the Extreme Male Brain theory of autism in half a million people. Proc Natl Acad Sci USA. 2018;115(48):12152–7.

Hain RDW. Voices of moral authority: parents, doctors and what will actually help. J Med Ethics. 2018;44(7):458.

Hain RDW. Parental discretion. Arch Dis Child. 2022;107:853.

Hain R. Critically ill children and the law: medical decision-making and the best interests principle. New Bioeth. 2024;31:67–71.

Hall B. The origin of parental rights. Public Aff Q. 1999;13(1):73–82.

Hare RM. Freedom and reason. Oxford: Oxford University Press; 1965.

Hare RM. When does potentiality count? A comment on Lockwood. Bioethics. 1988;2(3):214–26.

Harris J. The value of life. London: Routledge & Kegan Paul; 1985.

Harris J. Euthanasia and the value of life. In: Keown J, editor. Euthanasia examined: ethical, clinical and legal perspectives. Cambridge: Cambridge University Press; 1995.

Harrison H. Whey infant surgery without anesthesia went unchallenged. New York Times, 17 Dec 1987. p. A34.

Harrow Feen R. Abortion and exposure in ancient Greece. In: Bondeson WB, et al., editors. Abortion and the status of the fetus. Updated reprint with corrections ed. Lancaster: D. Reidel; 1983.

Hauerwas S. Suffering presence. Notre Dame: University of Notre Dame Press; 1986.

Hershenov DB, Hershenov RJ. If abortion, then infanticide. Theor Med Bioeth. 2017;38(5):387–409.

Hilarion. Oxyrhincus Papyrus 4.744.

Hoffmaster B. The rationality and morality of dying children. Hast Cent Rep. 2011;41(6):30–42.

Holm S. The peaceable pluralistic society and the question of persons. J Med Philos. 1988;13(4):379–86.

Hopwood N. Pictures of evolution and charges of fraud. Ernst Haeckel's embryological illustrations. Isis. 2006;97(2):260–301.

Hordern J. Compassion in healthcare. Oxford: Oxford University Press; 2020.

Howard H. The offence/defence of infanticide: a view from two perspectives. J Crim Law. 2018;82(6):470–81.

Hume D. Essays on suicide and the immortality of the soul. By the late David Hume, Esq. With remarks by the editor. To which are added, two letters on suicide, from Rousseau's Eloisa. A new ed. Basil: Collection of English Classics; 1799.

James W. The principles of psychology, Dover books on philosophy and psychology. Authorized ed. New York: Dover; 1950.

Johnson D. Putting a value on human and animal life. 2015. http://standpointmag.co.uk/dialogue-julyaugust11-putting-a-value-on-human-life-peter-singer-nigel-biggar-euthanasia-genocide-infanticide-animal-rights-huma#comment-25682. Accessed 2nd November.

Jones DG. The dead body as an object of investigation. In: Fitzgerald JJ, Moyse AJ, editors. Treating the body in medicine and religion: Jewish, Christian, and Islamic perspectives. 1st ed. London: Routledge; 2018.

Kant I, Abbott TK. Fundamental principles of the metaphysics of morals. Mineola: Dover Publications; 2005.

Kant I, Gregor M, Sullivan R. Metaphysics of morals (trans. Gregor M). Cambridge: Cambridge University Press; 1996.

Kant I, Wood AW, Schneewind JB. Groundwork for the metaphysics of morals, Rethinking the Western tradition. New Haven: Yale University Press; 2002.

King PO. Thomas Hobbes's children. In: Turner SM, Matthews GB, editors. The philosopher's child: critical perspectives in the Western tradition. Rochester/Woodbridge: University of Rochester Press; 1998.

Kirby L, et al. Rationing in the Pediatric Intensive Care Unit-ethical or unethical? Transl Pediatr. 2021;10(10):2836–44.

Koenigs M, et al. Damage to the prefrontal cortex increases utilitarian moral judgements. Nature. 2007;446(7138):908–11.

Krantz SF. Refuting Peter Singer's ethical theory: the importance of human dignity. Westport: Praeger; 2002.

Kuhse H. The sanctity-of-life doctrine in medicine: a critique. Oxford: Clarendon Press; 1987.

Kuhse H. Michael Tooley on possible people and promising. Camb Q Healthc Ethics. 1993;2(3):353–8.

L. Annaeus Seneca De Ira Liber 1. Ch. 15, sect 2.

Legrain L, Cleeremans A, Destrebecqz A. Distinguishing three levels in explicit self-awareness. Conscious Cogn. 2011;20(3):578.

Locke J. An essay concerning human understanding book II: ideas. Jonathan Bennett; 2004.

Lockwood M. Hare on potentiality: a rejoinder. Bioethics. 1988;2(4):343–52.

Long TA. Two philosophers in search of a contradiction: a response to Singer and Kuhse. J Med Ethics. 1990;16(2):95–6.

Lu M. Aristotle on abortion and infanticide. Int Philos Q. 2013;53(1):47–62.

Mampe B, et al. Newborns' cry melody is shaped by their native language. Curr Biol. 2009;19:1994–7.

Manson NC, O'Neill O. Rethinking informed consent in bioethics. Cambridge: Cambridge University Press; 2007.

Martin GB, Clark RD. Distress crying in neonates: species and peer specificity. Dev Psychol. 1982;18(1):3–9.

McGee A, Gardiner D. Differences in the definition of brain death and their legal impact on intensive care practice. Anaesthesia. 2019;74(5):569–72.

McGraw MB. Neural maturation as exemplified in the changing reactions of the infant to pin prick. Child Dev. 1941;12(1):31–42.

Messer N. Respecting life: theology and bioethics. London: SCM Press; 2011.

Mill JS. Utilitarianism. London: Longmans, Green and Co.; 1879.

Mill JS. A system of logic, ratiocinative and inductive: being a connected view of the principles of evidence and the methods of scientific investigation. Peoples ed. London: Longmans, Green, Reader, and Dyer; 1884.

Mill JS. Chapter V. Applications. In: Courtney WL, editor. On liberty. London and Felling-on-Tyne, New York and Melbourne: The Walter Scott Publishing Co., Ltd.; 1901.

Morin A. Self-recognition, theory-of-mind, and self-awareness: what side are you on? Laterality. 2011;16(3):367–83.

Mullin A. Children and the argument from 'marginal' cases. Ethical Theory Moral Pract. 2011;14(3):291–305.

Neuberger BJ, Guthrie LG, Aaronovitch D, Hameed K, Bonser T, Professor Lord Harries of Pentregarth, Charlesworth-Smith D, Professor Jackson E (2013), 'More care, less pathway: a review of the Liverpool Care Pathway', Independent Review of the Liverpool Care Pathway (Crown copyright).

Nye R. The child's curriculum. Oxford University Press; 2018.

O'Donovan O. Resurrection and moral order: an outline for evangelical ethics. 2nd ed. Leicester: William B. Eerdmans Pub. Co.; 1994.

O'Neill O. Autonomy and trust in bioethics, Gifford lectures. Cambridge: Cambridge University Press; 2002.

Pearsall P, Schwartz GER, Russek LGS. Changes in heart transplant recipients that parallel the personalities of their donors. Integr Med. 2000;2(2):65–72.

Peter LJ. Quotations for our time. London: Souvenir; 1996.

Pigliucci M. RS97 – Peter Singer on being a utilitarian in the real world. 2019. http://rationallyspeakingpodcast.org/show/rs97-peter-singer-on-being-a-utilitarian-in-the-real-world.html. Accessed 21 January.

Plunkett A, Parslow RC. Is it taking longer to die in paediatric intensive care in England and Wales? Arch Dis Child. 2016;101(9):798.

Popper KR, Eccles JC. The self and its brain. Berlin/London: Springer International; 1977.

Popper KR, Schilpp PA. The philosophy of Karl Popper, Library of living philosophers. La Salle: Open Court; 1974.

Price D. Lessons for health care rationing from the case of child B. BMJ. 1996;312(7024):167–9.

Rachels J. The end of life: euthanasia and morality, Studies in bioethics. Oxford: Oxford University Press; 1986.

Rachels J. Can ethics provide answers? And other essays in moral philosophy. Lanham/London: Rowman & Littlefield; 1997.

Ramsey P. The enforcement of morals: nontherapeutic research on children. Hast Cent Rep. 1976;6(4):21–30.

Ramsey P. The patient as person: explorations in medical ethics. Yale University Press; 2002.

Rawls J. A theory of justice. Cambridge, MA: Belknap Press of Harvard University Press; 1999.

Rennick JE, Childerhose JE. Redefining success in the PICU: new patient populations shift targets of care. Pediatrics. 2015;135(2):e289–91.

Richardson A. The politics of childhood: Wordsworth, blake, and catechistic method. ELH. 1989;56(4):853–68.

Rippon G. No, that study doesn't prove that men and women think differently. 2019. https://www. newstatesman.com/politics/feminism/2018/11/no-study-doesn-t-prove-men-and-women- think-differently. Accessed 24th June.

Rochat P. Five levels of self-awareness as they unfold early in life. Conscious Cogn. 2003;12(4):717–31.

Rochat P. The self as phenotype. Conscious Cogn. 2011;20(1):109–19.

Rochat P, Broesch T, Jayne K. Social awareness and early self-recognition. Conscious Cogn. 2012;21(3):1491–7.

Roma PG, et al. Mark tests for mirror self-recognition in capuchin monkeys (Cebus apella) trained to touch marks. Am J Primatol. 2007;69(9):989–1000.

Schapiro T. What is a child? Ethics. 1999;109(4):715–38.

Schneider C. The practice of autonomy: patients, doctors, and medical decisions. New York/ Oxford: Oxford University Press; 1998.

Sharkey K, Gillam L. Should patients with self-inflicted illness receive lower priority in access to healthcare resources? Mapping out the debate. J Med Ethics. 2010;36(11):661–5.

Sidgwick H. The complete works and select correspondence of Henry Sidgwick, Sidgwick, complete works and select correspondence. Charlottesville: InteLex Corporation; 1996.

Singer P. Famine, affluence and morality. Philos Public Aff. 1972;1(1):229–43.

Singer P. Bioethics and academic freedom. Bioethics. 1990;4(1):33–44.

Singer P. Animal liberation. 2nd ed. London: Pimlico; 1995.

Singer P. Practical ethics. New York: Cambridge University Press; 2011.

Singer P. Engaging with Christianity. In: Perry J, editor. God, the good, and utilitarianism: perspectives on Peter Singer. Cambridge: Cambridge University Press; 2014.

Sloane A. Singer, preference utilitarianism and infanticide. Stud Christ Ethics. 1999;12(2):47–73.

Smart B. Fault and the allocation of spare organs. J Med Ethics. 1994;20(1):26–30.

Sommers CH. Tooley's immodest proposal: abortion and infanticide. Hast Cent Rep. 1985;15(3):39–42.

Sorger B, et al. A real-time fMRI-based spelling device immediately enabling robust motor-independent communication. Curr Biol. 2012;22(14):1333–8.

Stevens JC. Must the bearer of a right have the concept of that to which he has a right? Ethics. 1984;95(1):68–74.

Taylor C. The language animal: the full shape of the human linguistic capacity. Cambridge, MA: The Belknap Press of Harvard University Press; 2016.

Tooley M. Abortion and infanticide. Philos Public Aff. 1972;2(1):37–65.

Traina CLH. Children and moral agency. J Soc Christ Ethics. 2009;29(2):19–37.

Trevarthen C, Aitken KJ. Infant intersubjectivity: research, theory, and clinical applications. J Child Psychol Psychiatry. 2001;42(1):3–48.

Tushnet M, Seidman LM. A comment on Tooley's abortion and infanticide. Ethics. 1986;96(2):350–5.

Tzourio-Mazoyer N, et al. Neural correlates of woman face processing by 2-month-old infants. NeuroImage. 2002;15(2):454–61.

Uleman JK. On Kant, infanticide, and finding oneself in a state of nature. Z Philos Forsch. 2000;54(2):173–95.

United Nations General Assembly. Convention on the Rights of the Child: adopted and opened for signature, ratification and accession by General Assembly resolution 44/25. Geneva: United Nations General Assembly; 1989.

Varelius J. The value of autonomy in medical ethics. Med Health Care Philos. 2006;9(3):377–88.

Varner, G.E. (2012), Personhood, ethics, and animal cognition: situating animals in Hare's two level utilitarianism (New York/Oxford: Oxford University Press).

Wall J. Ethics in light of childhood. Washington, DC: Georgetown University Press; 2010.

Wilkinson, D. (2013), Death or disability?: the 'Carmentis machine' and decision-making for critically ill children (Oxford: Oxford University Press).

Wilkinson D. In defense of a conditional harm threshold test for paediatric decision-making. In: Parental rights, best interests and significant harms: medical decision-making on behalf of children post Great Ormond St vs Yates. Oxford: Hart Publishing; 2019.

Williams BAO. A critique of utilitarianism. In: Smart JJC, Williams BAO, editors. Utilitarianism: for and against. Cambridge: Cambridge University Press; 1987.

Williamson L. Infanticide: an anthropological analysis. In: Kohl M, editor. Infanticide and the value of life. New York: Prometheus Books; 1978.

Wilson B, Hoffman J, Morgenstern J. Predictive inequity in object detection. arXiv:1902.11097. 2019. https://doi.org/10.48550/arXiv.1902.11097.

World Health Organization. Promoting rational use of medicines: core components. In: W.H.O. policy perspectives on medicines. Geneva: World Health Organization; 2002.

Wyatt J. Matters of life & death: human dilemmas in the light of Christian faith. Nottingham: Inter-Varsity Press; 2009.

Zweig A. Immanuel Kant's children. In: Turner SM, Matthews GB, editors. The philosopher's child: critical perspectives in the Western tradition. Rochester/Woodbridge: University of Rochester Press; 1998.

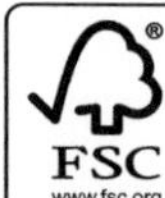